The Understanding of the

BRAIN

Second Edition

John C. Eccles
Professor Emeritus
State University of New York at Buffalo

based on
The Thirty-third Series of Lectures
on The Patten Foundation
delivered at the Bloomington Campus
Indiana University

McGraw-Hill Book Company
A Blakiston Publication

New York	St. Louis	San Francisco	Auckland
Düsseldorf	Johannesburg	Kuala Lumpur	London
Mexico	Montreal	New Delhi	Panama	Paris
São Paulo	Singapore	Sydney	Tokyo	Toronto

For Helena

The Understanding of the Brain

234567890 DODO 783210987

This book was set in Times Roman by Black Dot, Inc.
The editors were J. Dereck Jeffers and Richard Laufer;
the cover was designed by Nicholas Krenitsky;
the production supervisor was Thomas J. LoPinto.
R. R. Donnelley & Sons Company was printer and binder.

Library of Congress Cataloging in Publication Data

Eccles, John Carew, Sir.
    The understanding of the brain.

"A Blakiston publication."
    "Based on the thirty-third series of lectures of the
Pattern Foundation delivered at the Bloomington Campus,
Indiana University."
    Bibliography: p.
    Includes index.
    1. Brain. I. Title. [DNLM: 1. Brain—Physiology.
2. Neurophysiology. WL300 E17u]
QP376.E27   1977   612'.82   76-14941
ISBN 0-07-018865-3

Contents

Preface

Why did I give the title *The Understanding of the Brain* to this book? I am, of course, not claiming some final and complete understanding. That is indefinitely in the future, and may even be paradoxical: a brain completely understanding a brain. I undertake a much more modest task, namely to give an account of our present understanding, or, if you will, of my present understanding, because this is a personal communication. I venture to do this because, with the immense load of factual data, there is danger that those attracted to study brain research will not see the wood for the trees. To give an example of the explosive growth of reported information, the journal *Brain Research*, founded in 1966, published in one year (1975) 18 volumes totaling over 9000 pages; it is only one of the many journals started in the last few years.

Necessarily this personal communication will be somewhat biased in its treatment and in its emphasis. An overall review of brain research would entail multitudes of authors and multitudes of volumes if it were to cover all fields. Such handbooks do exist and more are being written. I assume nobody reads them through—rather their great value resides in their use as reference texts. I have written a book which can be read right through and which will give some vision of many aspects of brain research—of what I think are some of the ideas that are fundamental for the further ongoing enterprise of brain research, and also for the conceptual developments in the related disciplines of psychology and philosophy. Yet I have hopefully written a text which is so simple to read that it should be within the competence of a college student. In fact the book has gradually been formed by the many series of lectures I have given to college students and medical students. Nevertheless it also may be of help to those actually engaged in research in the brain sciences. I hope it may broaden their outlook on the problems of brain science and entice them to move into fields of research where there are problems that are most alluring and most rewarding.

So to sum up: this book is not to be regarded as a textbook or a reference book. Rather it is a personal communication in which I write about those aspects of the brain that are of particular interest to me and which I think are essential to any understanding of how the brain can carry out its marvellous and manifold functions.

I have been teaching for 50 years and what success I may have in communicating my ideas and my enthusiasm in this text is due to my efforts during all these years to improve my style of presentation. I have learned much from the responses and questions of my listeners. My gratitude is expressed in this book. I believe that we senior scientists have an obligation to communicate our scientific ideas to as wide an audience as possible. It is easy to talk in a technical language to the initiated; many do not try the exacting and vulnerable task of simplification, yet with preservation of the scientific character. By that I mean giving the sense of an ongoing scientific adventure—on the one hand creative imagination trying to create hypotheses beyond the known and on the other hand the rigorous testing of these hypotheses, these brain children, either to kill them, to change them, or to corroborate them, but never to give them a final accrediting or validation.

I believe that it is important to build up our story of the brain so that it relates to the human brain in the full range of its performance. Therein lies the greatest challenge. Marvellous as they are, the brains of invertebrates such as leeches, aplysia, or octopuses fail to be adequate models for man's brain with its abilities of conceptual thought, cognition, volition, and self-consciousness. Nevertheless investigations at these levels are of fundamental importance in that the unitary constituents and their simple intercommunications give the basis for understanding the units of higher brains and the properties of simple aggregates of these units. This also can be stated for investigations of the lower vertebrates. The importance of these studies of simpler nervous systems will be evident in this book. The major content of Chapters 1, 2, and 5 is concerned either with the invertebrate or the simpler vertebrate levels. Much more emphasis could have been placed upon the wonderful scientific investigations on these simpler nervous systems, but my aim was eventually to concentrate on more complex and more sophisticated brains.

In the chapter on the control of movement I have organized my account so that it relates to human movement, so far as this is possible. Finally in the last chapter, there has been a concentration on the human brain. I have there ventured into the intimidating realm of philosophy. I receive encouragement in this enterprise from distinguished philosophers who are peripheral to the modern guild of philosophers with their mystique of language and definition. I find the philosophical thought of these distinguished philosophers akin to mine. In particular I count myself fortunate beyond all measure to have the inspiration and guidance of Sir Karl Popper in my life when I am a scientist and when I am a scientist essaying paths in philosophy, as I do in the last chapter.

It is certainly unusual to have a book on the brain ascending from the simplest phenomena of the nervous system up to the role of the brain not only in cognition, creativity, volition, but also in relation to such themes as the nature of the conscious self, the role of language in the evolution both of the brain and of man's self-consciousness, and finally the problem of the meaning of life: the origin and destiny of the self-conscious being, unique and known only to the self that is at the core of being of each one of us.

We are only at the beginning of this great enterprise. I hope to have sketched in many of the important centers of present scientific understanding and to have given glimpses of what seem to be highly significant new developments. But it is a sketch and as such leaves out much detail. References are given after each chapter to guide further reading to fill in details and some of the gaps. At the end of the book there is a short list of general references that in many cases could serve for reference, but it is not suggested that the larger texts should be read through.

I recognize that large areas of the brain sciences are but cursorily treated, if treated at all. In particular neurochemistry is neglected, though not perhaps in its implications. My belief is that its period of greatness is yet to come—and it will be magnificent when we have precise chemical concepts accounting for all the information required to build a nervous system in all its detailed connectivity and to explain learning and all the ongoing trophic influences within neurons and between neurons, in fact for the whole content of Chapter 5. At another level neurochemistry is concerned with the nature of membranes, their structure, and their specific receptor properties related to the mode of operation of synaptic transmitter substances. Here neurochemistry links to neuropharmacology.

The immediate reason for writing this book was that I was invited to give the Patten Memorial Lectures of Indiana University at Bloomington during the spring of 1972. I worked for some months beforehand evolving the scope and the content of the six lectures. A particular requirement was the illustrations. Many new ones were constructed, but I drew heavily on the wide variety of excellent illustrations in the literature. The six lectures that I gave are reflected in the six chapters of this book. In order to preserve the quality of a personal communication, the lectures were recorded on tape and were then converted into a typescript by Mrs. Carol Shordone. The conversion to the present printed text proved to be an arduous undertaking—much more than I would have imagined, and the conversion had to be accompanied by a reduction in the number of illustrations which now amount to about three-fourths of the slides that were projected. However, I have hope that at the end of this long transmutation a written text will have been created that still carries the appeal of a personal communication in a lecture series. I might add here that I am deeply indebted to the enthusiastic audience that filled the large lecture hall to standing room for the whole series of six lectures. They were the most appreciative audience I have ever had. I tried to convey to them that the scientific study of the brain is an exciting experience, and that we are only at the beginning of this, the most wonderful adventure that man can undertake, since its aim is to understand man. As I have questioned above: How far will it be possible for us using our brains to understand our brains? And beyond that there is the problem of the self-conscious mind and its relationship to the brain, as briefly discussed in the last chapter.

Acknowledgments

I wish to express my thanks first to the Patten Foundation Committee and especially to my friend Professor Walter J. Moore for the invitation to give the Patten Lectures for the 1971–1972 academic year in the Bloomington Campus of Indiana University. My especial thanks go to the Chairman, Professor Richard Moody, for the excellence of all arrangements for the lectures and for the hospitality, in which Mr. Michael Waltz assisted so admirably.

I express my thanks to my wife, Helena, for her valuable comments on the manuscript and for composing many of the illustrations. I wish to give special thanks to the staff in my research unit for their devoted work—to my assistant, Miss Virginia Muniak, for the preparation of the manuscript in which she was assisted by Mrs. Mary Ann Davoli, and to Miss Tecla Rantucci for the preparation of many of the illustrations, and for the photography, in which she was assisted by Mr. Joseph Waldron.

Finally, I wish to express my grateful thanks to the many neuroscientists named below for so kindly allowing me to reproduce figures from their publications and for providing me with figures for reproduction: Lord Adrian, Doctors K. Akert, G. Allen, J. Altman, P. Andersen, H. Asanuma, R. Couteaux, D. R. Curtis, E. de Robertis, R. M. Eccles, E. V. Evarts, C. A. Fox, N. Geschwind, R. Granit, E. G. Gray, J. Hámori, H. K. Hartline, A. Hodgkin, D. Hubel, M. Jacobson, J. Jansen, H. H. Jasper, E. Kandel, B. Katz, H. H. Kornhuber, S. Kuffler, S. Landgren, B. Libet, T. Lømo, A. Lundberg, U. J. McMahan, P. B. C. Matthews, R. Miledi, S. Ochs, T. Oshima, W. Penfield, C. G. Phillips, R. Poritsky, G. Raisman, I. Rosén, N. H. Sabah, P. Scheid, P. Schiller, T. Sears, R. L. Sidman, A. Spencer, R. W. Sperry, J. Szentágothai, T. Thach, A. B. Vallbo, and T. Wiesel.

This work was supported by a grant from the National Institute of Neurobiological Diseases and Stroke, No. ROINB0822101, 2, 3.

The cover illustration is a simplified version of an aquarelle by Professor J. Szentágothai, and is here gratefully acknowledged. It represents a section of the cerebral cortex in perspective and corresponds in general with Fig. 4-6. The pyramidal cells are in red and all other cells in black.

John C. Eccles

Chapter 1

Neurons, Nerve Fibers, and the Nerve Impulse

INTRODUCTION

In Fig. 1-1 the brains of many vertebrates are drawn on the same scale. It gives us some concept of the way in which the brain has developed from fish, frog, turtle, pigeon, various mammals, and finally to the chimpanzee and man. The first point I want to make is that this is an evolutionary development over hundreds of millions of years; and the next point is that this human brain that does not look too distinguished on the outside, weighing about 1.5 kilograms (kg), is without any qualification the most highly organized and the most complexly organized matter in the universe.

Of course, the brains of higher animals are not greatly inferior in structure and in most aspects of operational performance—so far as we can yet determine—and some of them are many times larger. A whale's brain may weigh over 5 kg and would almost fill the lower part of the figure. Yet there is something very special about the human brain. It has a performance in relationship to culture, to consciousness, to language, to memory, that uniquely distinguishes it from even the most highly developed brains of other animals. That is a problem that we shall discuss

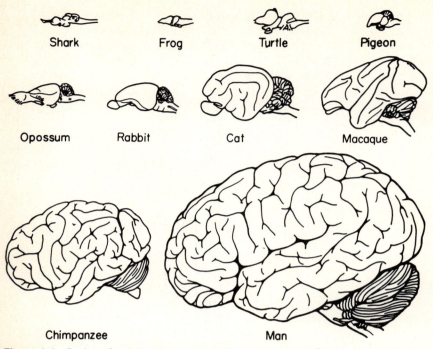

Shark   Frog   Turtle   Pigeon

Opossum   Rabbit   Cat   Macaque

Chimpanzee   Man

Figure 1-1   Brains of vertebrates drawn on the same scales. (*Courtesy of Professor J. Jansen.*)

in the last chapter. We shall see there that it is beyond our comprehension how these subtle properties of the conscious self came to be associated with a material structure, the human brain, that owes its origin to the biological process of evolution. I can state with complete assurance that for each of us our brains form the material basis of our experiences and memories, our imaginations, our dreams. Furthermore, it is through our brains that each of us can plan and carry out actions and so achieve expression in the world as, for example, I am doing now in expressing my ideas. I am able to do this because my stream of conceptual thinking can somehow or other activate neuronal changes that eventually result in all the complex movements that give writing. For each of us our brain is the material basis of our personal identity—distinguished by our selfhood and our character. In summary, it gives for each of us the essential "me." Yet when all this is said we are still only at the beginning of comprehending the mystery of what we are. This fundamental philosophical problem is still far beyond our understanding, though in the last chapter I will suggest that remarkable progress is being made in this, the greatest of all problems that confronts man. Essentially it is the problem formulated long, long ago and defined in the question of Plotinus, "What am I?"

Meanwhile, in the first five chapters I will be engaged in the task of trying to understand the nervous system as a neurobiologist. It is convenient at this stage to consider the brain as a machine, but it is a special kind of machine of a far higher order of complexity in perform-ance than any machine designed by man, even the most complex of computers. Please be warned against the claims of those computer devotees who seek to alarm us by their arrogant assertions that computers will soon outsmart man in all that matters. This is science fiction and these devotees are the modern variants of the idol makers of other superstitious ages; like them they seek power through the fostering of idolatry. But let me hasten to add that more than in any other science or technology we shall need advanced computer instrumentation in our scientific investiga-tions on the brain.

It will be my task first to describe the essential structure of the brain—the components from which it is built and how they are related to each other. Second, I will give an account of the mode of operation of the simplest components. Each of these two modes of investigation, the morphological, or structural, and the physiological, is complementary to the other and they form the basis of the third phase of my inquiry, which concerns the linkage of individual components into the simplest levels of organization. We are beginning to understand the simpler patterns of neuronal organization and the way they work. However, we are still at a very early stage of our attempt to understand the brain, which may well be the last of all the frontiers of knowledge that man can attempt to penetrate and encompass. I predict that it will occupy hundreds of years into the future. We will never run out of problems on this greatest of all problems confronting man because the problems multiply far faster than we solve them! Vigorous and exciting new disciplines emerge in such fields as neurochemistry, molecular neurobiology, neurogenetics, neuro-pharmacology, neuromathematics, and neurocommunications.

THE NEURON

To give you a first glimpse of a part of the brain, I show in Fig. 1-2*A* a low magnification of a histological section of a small segment of the human visual *cortex*. Each of these densely packed dots is a *neuron*, or *nerve cell*, and these are the individual components of which the whole brain is built. You have to imagine that the human cerebrum, shown in Fig. 1-1, has about 10,000 million of those little individual units. In Fig. 1-2*A* they are shown tightly packed together, but actually the density of the packing is much greater. In Fig. 1-2*A* only the bodies of the neurons are stained. You don't see all the interlacing branching structures stemming from each one of these cell bodies, as are shown in Fig. 1-2*B* for a few nerve cells. In this Golgi-stained section of the human cerebral cortex at about two times higher magnification you see one of those neurons (D) well displayed right in the center. Growing out upwards and sideways from the cell body there are several branching *dendrites*, as they are called, and projecting straight downwards is the fine *axon*, a *nerve fiber*. It gives a few branches before leaving the cortex, as also do the axons of cells B, C, E. Other neurons, A, F, J, K, in various shapes and sizes can be seen with their dendrites in different directions and with their axons branching and terminating in that section of the cerebral cortex.

The clarity of Fig. 1-2*B* depends on the fact that in this thin section only about 2 percent of the cells were stained by this special Golgi technique. Were it not for this lucky accident of random selection by the stain, which is still not understood, the composite of nerve cells seen in Fig. 1-2*A* with their dendrites and axons would be solid black, impenetrable to discrimination. This packing in the cerebral cortex is extremely dense and intricate, but we shall see that, despite this congestion, the neuronal components of the cortex or other regions of the brain are selectively connected to form organized patterns.

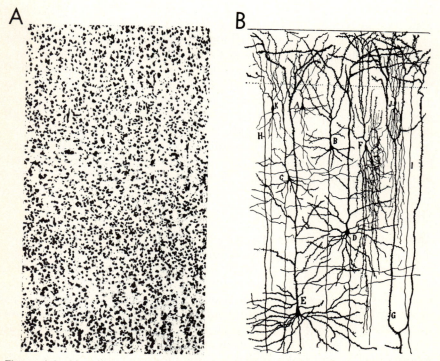

Figure 1-2 Magnified sections of cerebral cortex. In *A* all cell bodies are stained. (*From Sholl, 1956.*) *B* is a composite drawing of a Golgi preparation by Ramón y Cajal.

Diagrammatically the neuronal connectivity is indicated in the model of a neuron suitably enlarged in Fig. 1-3*A*. From the *soma*, or cell body, there are just the stumps of the dendrites which would be running a long way off in all directions, and projecting downwards from this soma there is the axon that eventually ends in many branches. The arrows show that messages or impulses come to the neuron by the many fine nerve fibers making contacts on the surface of the soma and dendrites. The sole output line is along the axon. Figure 1-3*B* shows the varieties of contacts made by nerve fibers on the dendrites and soma of a pyramidal cell of a special part of the cerebral cortex, which is similar to the pyramidal cells of Fig. 1-2*B*. Many contacts are made on small spines that branch out from the dendrites. Numerous small spines can be seen projecting from the dendrites of the cells in Fig. 1-2*B*.

It was first proposed by Ramón y Cajal, the great Spanish neuroanatomist, that the nervous system is made up of neurons which are isolated cells, not joined together in some syncytium, but each one independently

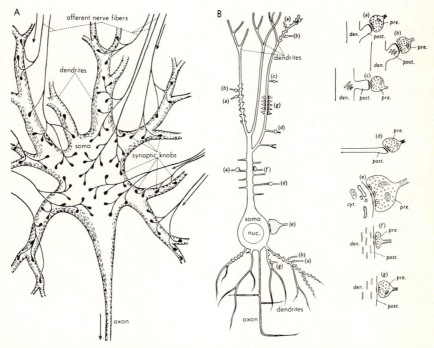

Figure 1-3 Synaptic endings on neurons. *A* is a general diagram, *B* is a drawing of a *hippocampal* pyramidal cell to illustrate the diversity of synaptic endings on the different zones of the apical and basal dendrites, and the inhibitory synaptic endings on the soma. The various types of synapses marked by the letters a to g are shown in detail to the right. [*L. H. Hamlyn, J. Anat., 97: (1963).*]

living its own biological life. This concept is called the *neuron theory*. How then does a neuron receive information from other nerve cells? This happens by means of these fine branches of the axons of the other neurons that make contact with its surface and end in little knobs scattered all over its soma and dendrites as indicated in Fig. 1-3*A* and *B*. It was Sherrington's concept that these contact areas are specialized sites of communication, which he labeled *synapses* from the Greek word *synapto*, which means "to clasp tightly." In Fig. 1-3*A* we can recognize the *afferent fibers* terminating in the *synaptic knobs* on the *soma* and the many *dendrites* of the *neuron* with the single *axon* leaving from its base. These are all basic words.

The synaptic knobs cover the surface far more densely than is shown in Fig. 1-3*A*. For example, in the reconstruction of Fig. 1-4*A* a *synaptic scale* provides an almost complete coverage of the surfaces of the soma, the dendritic stumps, and even the axonal origin. On the axon there is shown the beginning of the myelin sheath that will be discussed later in this chapter. When the synaptic knobs are highly magnified by electron microscopy (Fig. 1-4*B*), their location at the ends of fine nerve fibers (Fig. 1-3*A*) is not usually shown, but they can be seen to be separated from the surface of the dendrite by an extremely narrow space. This *synaptic cleft*, as it is called, completely separates the nerve terminal from the cell surface. The neuron theory of Cajal is thus corroborated. The whole communication apparatus, the knobs, the space, and the subjacent neuronal surface, was named the *synapse* by Sherrington, and the derivative terms are *synaptic knob* and *synaptic cleft*. Synapses such as those of Fig. 1-4*B* are the structural basis of the chemical transmission whereby the messages that come down the fine fibers to synaptic knobs on the recipient cell act on that cell by means of the secretion of minute amounts of specific chemical substances. The mode of operation of synapses will be described in Chaps. 2 and 3.

In Figs. 1-3*B* and 1-4*A*, synapses are seen to vary widely in size, which is in agreement with the recent electron-microscopic observations of Conradi, who describes five types of synapses on motoneurons. The very large synapses (Fig. 1-4*A*) presumably are the endings from afferents of annulospiral endings giving the monosynaptic excitation that is dia-

Figure 1-4 Synapses on surface of motoneurons. *A*. Reconstruction from serial electron micrographs of motoneuron with its highly packed surface scale of synaptic knobs (boutons), some being large. [*Poritsky, J. Comp. Neurol.,* **135:**423–452 (1969).] *B*. Electron micrograph of two synaptic knobs on a motoneuron in a fish spinal cord; that to the left is excitatory with spherical vesicles (rv) and dense staining on each side of the synaptic cleft (sc), and that to the right is inhibitory with ellipsoid vesicles (fv) and a much lighter staining of the membranes on each side of the synaptic cleft. Mitochondria are labeled m. *(From Gray, 1970.)*

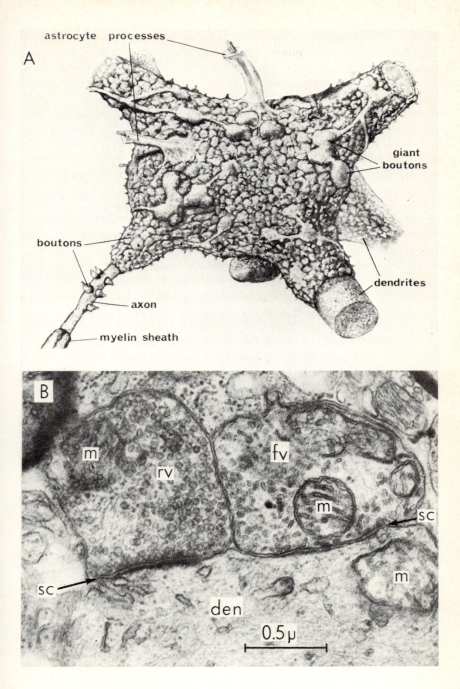

grammed in Fig. 1-6A, and on them Conradi finds small synaptic knobs, which form a distinctive type of synapse that will be referred to in Chap. 3 (Fig. 3-12). Figure 1-4A gives some concept of the busy life that a nerve cell has with incessant bombardment by impulses activating its dense coverage by synapses, which even are on the axon at its origin. However, we shall see that the neuron has some relief because, as first recognized by Sherrington, many of these synapses, the *inhibitory synapses*, are specialized to prevent the neuron from firing impulses in response to the *excitatory synapses*. The neuron is in the hands, as it were, of the two opposing operations of excitation and inhibition, which is the theme of much of Chap. 3. Meanwhile it can be noted that it is now possible to identify these two classes of synapses in electron micrographs, as is diagrammatically shown in Fig. 1-4B. The synapse to the left is excitatory with numerous spherical *synaptic vesicles* and that to the right is inhibitory with fewer vesicles of ellipsoid shape.

By means of the freeze-etch technique, Akert and associates have examined the inner and outer aspects of the surface membrane surrounding a synaptic knob. The cutaway-perspective drawing of Fig. 1-5 shows

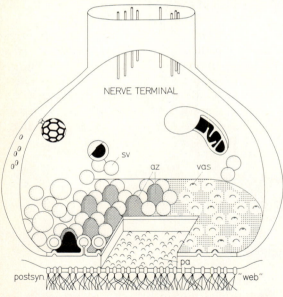

Figure 1-5 Schema of the mammalian central synapse. The active zone (az) is more complex and allows far more vesicle attachment sites (vas) per square unit of surface than the motor endplate. The postsynaptic aggregation of intramembranous particles is restricted to the area facing the active zone. The connection between the particles and the "web" of De Robertis (1964) is hypothetical. sv is synaptic vesicles, pa is particle aggregations on postsynaptic membrane (postsyn.). (*Akert, Peper, and Sandri, 1975.*)

that the synaptic vesicles (sv) tend to be in an hexagonal array separated by dense structures. To the right there has been removal by the etch technique of the vesicles and dense structures, so disclosing the underlying small protuberances (vas) into the synaptic knob from the synaptic cleft. These correspond to the attachment sites of the vesicles through which they may discharge their contents into the synaptic cleft. Below there is a cutaway area of the knob revealing the outer face of the postsynaptic membrane encrusted with fine particles (pa) which may be the postsynaptic receptor sites (cf. Fig. 2-10). This illustration gives some indication of the cellular machinery associated with the movement and discharge of synaptic vesicles and with the postsynaptic action of the transmitter, but the mode of operation of this machinery is as yet unknown. Similar fine structures occur at the neuromuscular junction, but there the synaptic vesicle attachment sites are arranged in bands that are congruent with the folds on the postsynaptic membrane (cf. Fig. 2-2B).

A nerve cell is filled with structures called organelles that are the basis of the biochemical processes associated with its extremely high metabolism: mitochondria, endoplasmic reticulum, ribosomes, etc. Nerve cells can be considered as cauldrons of metabolic activity. They have one of the highest metabolic rates of mammalian cells and have very specialized chemical enzyme systems. This intense metabolism is required for operating the ionic pumps across the surface membrane so as to maintain the correct ionic composition inside the cell (cf. Fig. 1-13), and it is also required for the manufacture of the chemical transmitting substances (cf. Fig. 2-10B) and for the manufacture and transport of specific substances along the axon that we shall be considering in Chap. 5. These various activities will be discussed later in this chapter and in the next four chapters.

SIGNALING BY NERVE IMPULSES

You now have some concept of what a neuron is in itself. Now we come to consider how they are concerned in receiving and giving signals. In Fig. 1-6A, below the diagram of the spinal cord, there is a muscle which has a stretch receptor, or *annulospiral ending* (cf. Fig. 3-1A). When you give a brief pull to a muscle, as when you make a knee jerk, impulses run up in the *primary afferent fibers* from the stretch receptors and excite nerve cells in the spinal cord (the so-called *motoneurons*) which fire impulses out to the muscles that are so made to contract. That's a knee jerk. It is the very simplest *central reflex pathway*, and we will be dealing with it in Chap. 3. My purpose now is to remind you that the nervous system receives signals from receptors such as from this one in muscle (cf. Fig. 1-8A). In Fig. 1-6B there is shown diagrammatically to the right a

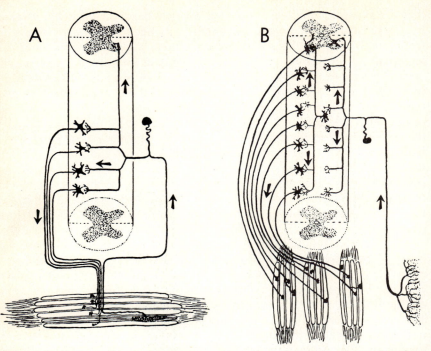

Figure 1-6 Reflex pathways for monosynaptic reflex arc. *A*, with afferent fiber from annulospiral ending, and for polysynaptic flexor reflex (*B*) with cutaneous afferent fiber. The three muscles in *B* represent flexors of hip, knee, and ankle. (*Modified from Ramón y Cajal, 1909.*)

cutaneous receptor that is excited by touch or pressure or irritation on the skin (Fig. 1-7*A*). The impulses run up the primary afferent fiber into the spinal cord, then via an *interneuron* to motoneurons and so to the flexor muscles that bend joints; three such muscles are shown. The resulting *flexor reflex* withdraws the limb from the irritating stimulus.

On the surface of the hairy skin of a cat there are very sensitive *tactile receptors* like that shown in Fig. 1-6*B*. In Fig. 1-7*A* steady indentations of the indicated amounts are put upon such a tactile receptor, causing impulses to be discharged along its nerve fiber, which are seen as brief potentials. With 88 microns (μm) the receptor fires fast at the start, then it slows up but keeps going during the indentation. This same fast-slowing sequence can be seen with the larger indentations—154, 374, and 706 μm. The receptor is firing more frequently the stronger the indentation. This is a typical signal system. All our touch sensations come like this from special cutaneous receptors firing along the primary nerve fibers. In Fig. 1-7*A* it will be seen that all of the impulses have the same size. With stronger indentation there is a faster train of them. It is a

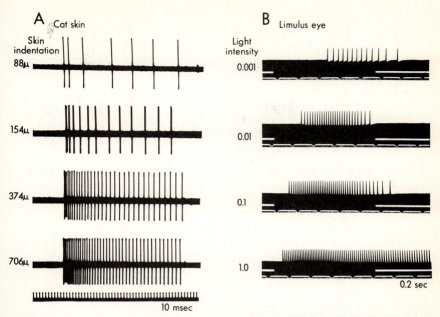

Figure 1-7   Impulse discharges from receptor organs. *A.* Tactile receptor of cat hairy skin discharging into a single afferent fiber in response to the indicated skin indentations. *(From Mountcastle, 1966.) B.* Photoreceptor of limulus eye discharging into a single afferent fiber in response to a 1-s flash of light signaled by the gap in the white bar and of indicated intensity. [*H. K. Hartline, J. Cell. Comp. Physiol.,* **5:**229 *(1934)*.]

universal property of the nervous system that signaling is coded by information like this. *Trains of similarly sized impulses signal intensity by frequency.* It is like a Morse code with dots only.

In Fig. 1-7*B* you see discharges from a quite different receptor, a light receptor in the eye of an invertebrate. When the intensities of light increase by factors of 10, that single unit fires more and more frequently. Again intensity is coded by frequency and the discharges always have the same size. In Fig 1-8*A*, pull upon a muscle excites a stretch receptor (AS in Fig. 3-1*A*) that discharges during the whole duration of the stretch. Some receptors, called *phasic,* only fire at the onset of the stimulus. Others, as in Figs. 1-7 and 1-8*A*, discharge throughout the whole duration of an applied stimulus and are called *tonic.* There are all varieties in between.

The same general principle of signaling occurs on the output side of the nervous system to muscles. For example, in Fig. 1-8*B* the firing of a motoneuron to an eye muscle is associated with a downward movement of the eye, which is signaled by the lower trace. A wide range of

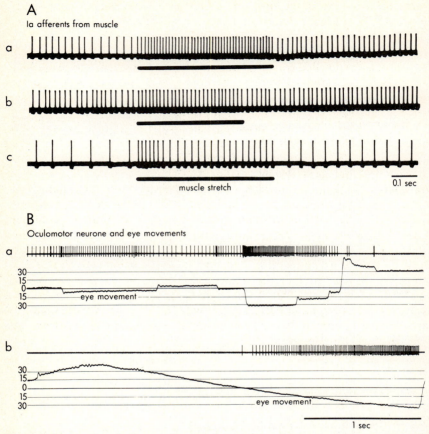

Figure 1-8 Impulse discharges from and to muscle. *A* . Discharges of impulses from an annulospiral ending of cat soleus muscle in response to a slow stretch (2.9 mm/s) during the bars. The muscle spindle was under strong influence from γ-motoneuron discharge (cf. Fig. 4-7) in a, less in b, and zero in c. [*J. K. S. Jansen and P. B. C. Matthews, J. Physiol.*, **161**:357 (1962).] *B*. In upper traces are discharges from an oculomotor neuron of a cat and in lower traces are the simultaneously recorded eye movements given in degrees of angle up or down. [*P. H. Schiller, Exp. Brain Res.*, **10**:347 (1970).]

frequencies of impulse discharge is related to the amount of downward eye movement. With strong upward movement the motoneuron is silent. Note in *b* that the discharge begins at about position 0 and progressively increases with further downward movement.

Throughout the whole central nervous system—with the complexities of organization suggested in Figs. 1-2 and 1-3—*the signaling is by coded information of uniformly sized impulses.* Intensity is signaled by frequency as in Figs. 1-7 and 1-8. I like discussing this problem of impulse coding because in recent years my research has been based on the firing patterns of single nerve cells that have this coded language in all their responses to controlled sensory inputs. In this way we learn to understand the mode of operation of some parts of the brain. In fact, nerve impulses are the only language that is used in the brain for communication at a distance.

All peripheral receptor organs generate the firing of impulses along the nerve fiber that projects from them by reducing the electrical potential across the surface membrane of the terminals of that afferent nerve fiber—a process called *depolarization.* This has been established by most thorough investigations on many species of receptor organs, though the retina is an exception, but their consideration is beyond the scope of these chapters. Figure 1-9 illustrates an elegant model of receptor organ action. A single nerve fiber (a crab axon) is subjected to steady electric currents of relative intensities as indicated. At a threshold strength (1.00) there is a slow firing during the whole duration of the current. As the current intensity is increased, there is an increase in frequency. Again, intensity is signaled as frequency. This is the basic mode of signaling in the nervous system, both central and peripheral. It was for his fundamental contributions to the understanding of nerve impulse signaling that Adrian was awarded the Nobel prize in 1932.

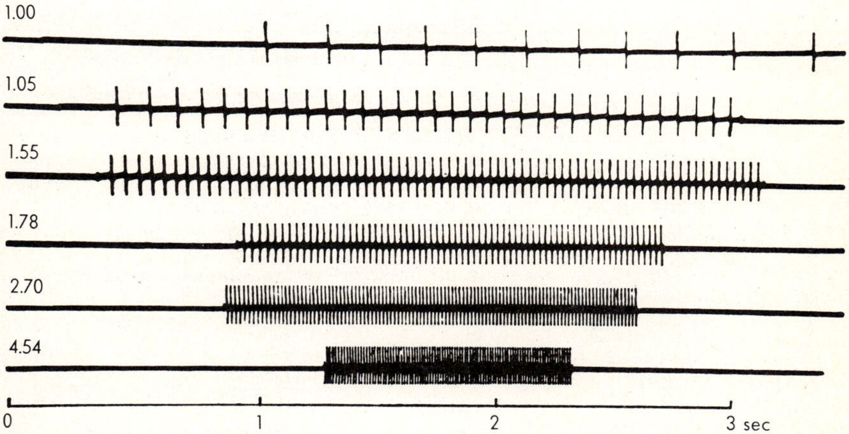

Figure 1-9   Repetitive responses of a single nerve fiber of a crab nerve in response to a constant depolarizing current, the on and off being signaled by slight artifacts. Current strengths are given relative to threshold. [*A. L. Hodgkin, J. Physiol., **107**:165 (1948).*]

THE NERVE IMPULSE

We now come to the question, What is this impulse that is the basis of all signaling? We have regarded it so far as an extremely brief message that runs along the nerve fibers. The frequency of firing may be at a higher or lower frequency, but the impulse is always of the same size. It is the universal currency of the nervous system. It is the only currency that the nervous system knows for any actions at a distance. All signals from one nerve cell to another are conveyed by impulses. A nerve cell not firing impulses is mute. It is not communicating. There are a few minor exceptions to this generalization with action at short distances. They will be referred to in the third chapter (cf. Fig. 3-15).

In experimental efforts to study the nature of the nerve impulse the giant axon of the squid has been of inestimable value. It has been known since the 1930s and has been utilized enormously, most fruitfully by Hodgkin and Huxley, for which they received the Nobel prize in 1963. Figure 1-10 shows a squid with its tentacles. From the stellate ganglion several nerves run out to the mantle musculature conveying impulses that bring about its contraction. Contraction of the mantle powerfully ejects water, and the squid jets in the reverse direction (to the left in Fig. 1-10*A*), a true jet propulsion! When you look at one of those mantle nerves from

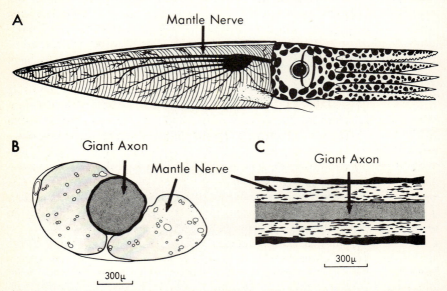

Figure 1-10 Drawings showing squid with the mantle nerves radiating from its stellate ganglion. In the transverse and longitudinal sections the single giant axon is seen embedded in the mantle nerve.

the stellate ganglion in section, the most prominent feature is the giant axon, which is almost 500 μm across in Fig. 1-10*B*. In the longitudinal section (Fig. 1-10*C*) the giant axon is seen to run straight and to have smooth walls, so they can be easily isolated by dissection to give a beautifully clean axon. It turns out that this giant axon has all the properties, essentially, of our own nerve fibers, and because of its enormous size it can be investigated much more effectively.

In Fig. 1-10*B* and *C* it appears that the fiber has a uniform core surrounded by a thin membrane. When studied by electron microscopy, the essential part of the membrane is only 70 angstroms (Å) thick (1 Å is 10^{-10} meter), so it is very tenuous indeed. The content of the axon has the consistency of a jelly, and for most purposes you can substitute an appropriate salt solution without deteriorating impulse conduction by the fiber. For example, Baker and Shaw were able to squeeze out the contents of the giant axon with an open end by a kind of microroller, leaving a collapsed, flattened axon that appeared destroyed. Yet, when they reinflated it by an appropriate salt solution (a potassium salt) the fiber was restored and conducted well for hours. The refill should be isotonic and with the normal high potassium for its cationic content, but the anion is unimportant.

Figure 1-11 illustrates a simple yet fundamental experiment on a single giant axon immersed in a salt solution resembling the blood of the squid. The axon (black) is shown in two segments so as to indicate a long distance between the stimulating and recording electrodes. As I mentioned earlier, stimulation by an electric current is effective when it takes charge off the membrane, depolarizing it and so setting up impulses, as in that crab axon of Fig. 1-9 that fired repetitively during a long current. Instead, in Fig. 1-11, a brief current was applied through the stimulating electrode just on the surface of the axon. In the trace below the diagram when the recording microelectrode was outside, there was zero potential against the indifferent electrode; then suddenly, as the recording electrode was advanced to penetrate the membrane, there appeared a membrane potential of −80 millivolts (mV), which is the voltage across the surface membrane from inside to outside. This immediate change is quite dramatic. Though the microelectrode has a tip diameter of less than 1 μm, it can be either outside or inside because the membrane is only 70 Å, which is only about 1 percent of the tip diameter.

In Fig. 1-11, after intracellular recording had been established, the first three applied currents were in the direction to increase the membrane potential. Even quite a large current had no effect except for the brief downward artifacts that are seen to grade with the intensity of the current. With the reverse direction the two weakest currents also were ineffective, but, at a certain intensity of the brief depolarizing current, a

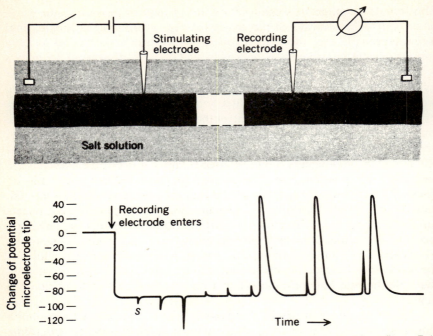

Figure 1-11 Method of stimulating and recording with a single giant fiber. Full description in text. (*From Katz, 1966.*)

full-sized impulse was recorded—nothing less. With two further increases in the applied currents there was no increase in the response, only in the artifact. This is a good illustration of the all-or-nothing nature of the response. The explanation will be given later. Already we have seen examples of all-or-nothing impulses in Figs. 1-7, 1-8, and 1-9. In fact, all that can be propagated along an axon is a response that is full-sized for the condition of that axon. The alternative is nothing. And this sharp antithesis holds whether the axon is fired by receptors (Figs. 1-7 and 1-8A), or by nerve cells (Fig. 1-8B) or by stimulating electrodes (Figs. 1-9 and 1-11).

A further important discovery is illustrated in Fig. 1-11. During the impulse the membrane potential does not just go up to zero; it attains 30 mV or more in reverse. This discovery in 1939 by Hodgkin, Huxley, and Cole falsified all the theories up to that time about the nature of the impulse, which was thought to arise as a brief removal of the membrane charge. The observed reversal gave rise to most interesting investigations. The impulse became a more complicated phenomenon than had been thought. The elegant biological mechanism that was disclosed in the subsequent investigations can only be understood in terms of the nature of the surface membrane of the nerve fiber and of the ionic concentration differences across it.

THE SURFACE MEMBRANE OF NERVE FIBERS AND NERVE CELLS

In the light of intensive investigations the very thin membrane around the nerve fiber and nerve cell can be pictured as in Fig. 1-12. The main components of the 70-Å membrane are arranged as a bimolecular leaflet of phospholipid molecules, with hydrophilic polar groups pointing both outwards and inwards. Such membranes can be made artificially and in many of their properties the artificial membranes resemble natural cell membranes. In addition protein molecules are associated with the membrane. Some on the inner and outer surfaces give the membrane stability. Some proteins make ensembles across the membrane that can be the basis of channels for ion penetration; one is shown to the right. In addition there are specific proteins on the outer side of the membrane that give it the specific properties described in Chap. 5 (Fox, 1972; Reisfeld and Kahan, 1972).

In the first place it will be realized that the bimolecular phospholipid leaflet is very highly resistant to electric current and has the considerable capacity of about 1 microfarad (μF) per square centimeter (cm^2), a value that accords with a dielectric coefficient of 5 and a plate separation of 50

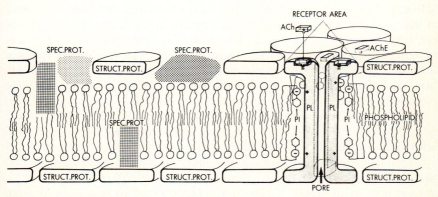

Figure 1-12 Macromolecular organization of surface membrane. The basic structure is a bimolecular leaflet of phospholipid molecules that is stabilized by structural proteins (Struct. Prot.) applied to both surfaces. In addition there are various specific proteins (Spec. Prot.) or other macromolecules applied to the outer surface or penetrating through the membrane. Finally, a transmembrane pore is shown with controls by receptor sites for acetylcholine (ACh) (cf. Figs. 2-10 and 2-11). (*Modified from De Robertis, 1971.*)

Å. The surface membrane of the giant axon may be likened to a wrapping around it of a leaky condenser, with a resistance of 1000 ohm-cm^2, because ions pass through the many channels across the membrane that are occupied by proteins.

The surface membranes of all nerve fibers and nerve cells have essentially the same structure and properties throughout the whole of the invertebrate and vertebrate kingdoms. The cell membrane was a basic innovation at a very early stage of evolution, and it was such a good discovery that it can be seen to be essentially the same over a wide range of invertebrates and with all vertebrates. Furthermore, the impulse itself was also a very early innovation and in its essentials it has been preserved right up to the vertebrates and the mammals. No engineer could design or imagine anything so beautiful and efficient and effective as a nerve impulse and the communication that it gives along nerve fibers, and so from one nerve cell to others.

I will use the mammalian nerve cell for exposition because the theme of this book is the mammalian and, especially, the human brain. As shown in Fig. 1-13A the surface membrane of a nerve cell separates two aqueous solutions that have very different ionic compositions. The external concentrations are approximately the same as for a protein-free filtrate of blood plasma. The internal concentrations are derived more indirectly from investigations of the equilibrium potentials for some physiological processes that are specifically produced by one or two ion species. Within the cell, sodium and chloride ions are at a lower concentration than on the outside, the ratios being about 10:1 and 14:1. With potassium there is an even greater disparity—almost 30-fold—but in the reverse direction. Under resting conditions potassium and chloride ions move through the membrane much more readily than sodium. Necessarily the electrical potential across the membrane influences the rates of diffusion of charged particles between the inside and outside of the cell. The potential across the surface membrane is normally about -70 mV, the minus sign signifying inside negativity, as demonstrated in Fig. 1-11.

The equilibrium potentials in Fig. 1-13A are derived from the concentrations by the Nernst equation. This equation simply gives the electrical potential that just balances a concentration difference of charged particles, such as ions, so that there is equality in their inward and outward diffusion rates across the membrane.

In Fig. 1-13C there is shown across the membrane a large electrochemical potential difference for sodium ions (130 mV) which is derived from 70 mV for the membrane potential plus 60 mV from the concentration difference as calculated by the Nernst equation. This large electrochemical gradient causes the inward diffusion of sodium ions to be more than 100 times faster than outwards. Fortunately the resting membrane is much more impermeable to sodium ions than to potassium and chloride

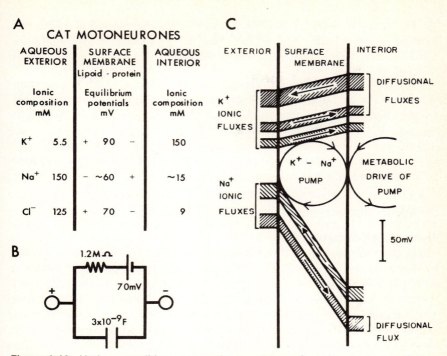

A

CAT MOTONEURONES

AQUEOUS EXTERIOR	SURFACE MEMBRANE Lipoid - protein	AQUEOUS INTERIOR
Ionic composition mM	Equilibrium potentials mV	Ionic composition mM
K$^+$ 5.5	+ 90 –	150
Na$^+$ 150	– ~60 +	~15
Cl$^-$ 125	+ 70 –	9

B

1.2MΩ

70mV

3x10^{-9}F

C

EXTERIOR   SURFACE MEMBRANE   INTERIOR

K$^+$ IONIC FLUXES

Na$^+$ IONIC FLUXES

K$^+$ – Na$^+$ PUMP

DIFFUSIONAL FLUXES

METABOLIC DRIVE OF PUMP

50mV

DIFFUSIONAL FLUX

Figure 1-13 Various conditions across the membrane of a cat motoneuron. *A* gives approximate ionic compositions inside and outside and the respective equilibrium potentials. *B* is a formal electrical model for an average motoneuron as measured by a microelectrode in the soma. *C* shows ionic fluxes across the membrane for K and Na ions under resting conditions. These fluxes are in part diffusional down the electro-chemical gradients as indicated, and in part due to specific ion pumps driven by metabolism. The fluxes due to diffusion and the operation of the pump are distinguished by the cross-hatching, and the magnitudes are given by the respective widths of the channels. (*From Eccles, 1957.*)

ions, else the cell would be rapidly swamped with sodium ions. But of course there must be some other factor concerned in balancing sodium transport across the membrane even at an unbalanced slow diffusion rate. This is accomplished by a kind of pump that uses metabolic energy to force sodium ions uphill (up the electrochemical gradient) and so outward through the cell membrane, as is diagrammatically shown in Fig. 1-13*C*. This diagram further shows that there is an excess of diffusion outwards of potassium down the electrochemical gradient of about 20 mV for potassium, and again the transport of potassium ions is balanced by an inward pump. In fact, as shown, the sodium and potassium pumps are loosely coupled together and driven by the same metabolic process.

With the squid axon all ionic concentrations are several times larger, because they are isotonic with the sea water in which the animal lives;

nevertheless the ratios are similar, being for inside/outside, 20:1 for potassium, 1:9 for sodium, and 1:14 for chloride. Thus the diagrammatic representations in Fig. 1-13C may be assumed also for the squid axon, both for electrochemical gradients and for ionic fluxes.

As shown in the formal electrical diagram of Fig. 1-13B, under resting conditions the surface membrane of the nerve cell and its axon resembles a leaky condenser charged at a potential of about -70 mV (inside to outside). If this charge is suddenly diminished by about 20 mV, i.e., to -50 mV, there is a sudden further change in the membrane potential—a nerve impulse has been generated as in Fig. 1-11. We will now consider the essential ionic mechanisms.

THE IONIC MECHANISM OF THE NERVE IMPULSE

The ionic mechanism of the impulse is essentially shown in Fig. 1-14, where the time scale is in thousandths of second (s) or milliseconds (ms). To the right is the membrane potential scale showing that the resting potential is about -65 mV. The time course of the membrane potential change during the impulse is given by the broken line (V) rising up to a reversal potential of almost $+30$ mV and then rapidly coming down again. The explanation of this sequence of potential changes is provided by the measured time courses of the changes in the sodium and potassium conductances (see scale to left) across the membrane (g_{Na} and g_K).

This explanation is based upon the investigations by Hodgkin, Huxley, Katz, and Keynes on the squid giant axon using such refined techniques as voltage clamping of the membrane and measurements of ionic fluxes by radiotracers. These investigations have been carried out under conditions where the internal and external ionic concentrations have been widely varied. For a full description of these elegant investigations reference should be made to Hodgkin's book *The Conduction of the Nervous Impulse*.

In Fig. 1-14 the sodium conductance (g_{Na}) is initially so dominant that the membrane potential (V) approaches by an extremely steep rise the sodium equilibrium potential (V_{Na}) at about $+50$ mV. However, quite quickly the potential ceases to rise and then falls toward the initial resting level. This occurs for two reasons. First, even if the membrane potential is clamped at a depolarized level, the sodium conductance is quite transient, rapidly declining to the very low level of the resting state. More important is the increase in potassium conductance (g_K) that begins a little later than the increase in g_{Na} and runs a slower time course. The large membrane potential change during the impulse (V) moves the membrane far from the equilibrium potential for potassium ions (V_K at about -75 mV in Fig. 1-14), so establishing a high gradient for the *outward* flux of

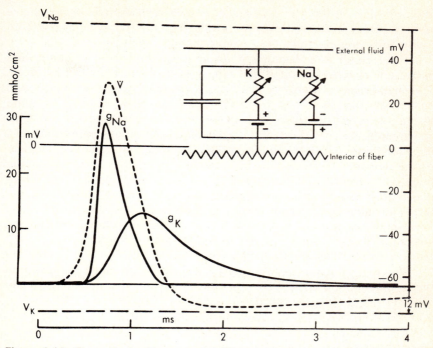

Figure 1-14 Theoretical action potential (V) and membrane conductance changes (g_{Na} and g_K) obtained by solving the equations derived by Hodgkin and Huxley for the giant axon of the squid at 18.5°C. V_{Na} and V_K are the equilibrium potentials for sodium and potassium across the membrane. The inset shows an element of the excitable membrane of a nerve fiber. Note the constant capacity, the channel for K, and the channel for Na. [*Modified from A. L. Hodgkin and A. F. Huxley, J. Physiol., 117:23 (1952).*]

potassium ions across the membrane and counteracting the effect of the sodium influx. At first it slows, then checks the rise of the potential (V) and then it causes it to fall to the initial level and even reverses it for some milliseconds. Meanwhile this restoration of the resting membrane potential has accomplished the turning down of both g_{Na} and g_K to their resting levels. The depolarization of the impulse (V) occupies only about 1 ms in Fig. 1-14, but for a mammalian nerve cell or fiber the changes are still faster, an impulse having a total duration of only 0.5 ms.

The inset diagram of Fig. 1-14 shows an electrical model of the sodium and potassium conductances across the membrane with the capacity also shown as in Fig. 1-13B. The essential mechanism concerned in the rising phase of the impulse is a kind of autocatalyzing reaction. An initial depolarization leads to an increase in sodium conductance and that in turn leads to entry of sodium and that to more depolarization, and so on up to the peak of the impulse. This explains why the impulse is all-or-nothing. It is the product of a self-regenerative or explosive reaction. Once it starts, it rises to its full effect, the energy being provided by the ions running down their electrochemical gradients.

Figure 1-15 is a diagram of an impulse showing the sodium and potassium channels through the membrane with their control by gates. The membrane is shown with separate channels for the sodium and potassium ions, because these channels and their gates have quite distinctive properties. They key convention is given in the inset. To give an example, not only do the gates open at different times in response to a depolarization (Fig. 1-14) but the sodium channels are selectively blocked by the poison TTX (tetrodotoxin) when applied on the outside, while the potassium channels are selectively blocked by TEA (tetraethylammonium) injected on the inside. There are various other distinctions between them, so they are depicted as separate channels with their own gates. Presumably each species of channel is some specific protein and enzyme structure across the membrane resembling that shown in Fig. 1-12 intercepting the bimolecular leaflet.

Figure 1-15 shows that at a certain stage of membrane depolarization the sodium gates open widely in the autocatalyzed reaction already

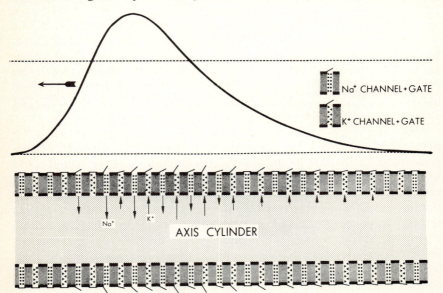

Figure 1-15 Opening of sodium and potassium gates at an instant during the propagation of a nerve impulse. In the upper part of the diagram there is a plot of the membrane potential along the fiber, showing reversal as in Fig. 1-14. In the lower part the opening of the two species of gates is symbolically represented by the angles of the respective gates. The thicknesses of the membranes on either side are greatly exaggerated with respect to the axis cylinder.

described and then rapidly close. The potassium gates begin to open a little after the sodium gates are fully opened during the falling phase of the impulse. Their full closure is seen to be delayed until after the end of the impulse, as in Fig. 1-14.

Recent work by Armstrong, Keynes, and their associates on the squid axon shows that the opening of the sodium gates is associated with an outward capacitative current across the membrane. This is called the *gating current*. This is a very small and brief effect (about 200 μs in duration). It can be recognized only when the resultant sodium currents are reduced to zero by TTX and the absence of external sodium. Closing of the sodium gates is associated with the reverse current. It is possible to estimate the number of sodium gates as being almost 500 per μm^2. This figure is in good agreement with the density determined for these gates by tritiated TTX. There is as yet no evidence that there is a related process for potassium gates, though its existence is theoretically predictable.

THE CONDUCTION OF THE NERVE IMPULSE

Now we are in the position to answer the question, How does the impulse travel along the fiber? So far we have considered in detail the happenings in one segment of the nerve fiber as the nerve impulse passes along it. The scale of Fig. 1-14 is in milliseconds. Figures 1-15 and 1-16A are diagrams with a scale in length, not time. In Fig. 1-16A the axon is shown in longitudinal section w1th the charge across the membrane (negativity inwards) ahead of the impulse and the reversal of charge during the impulse brought about by the influx of sodium. Later the efflux of potassium restores the charge.

When we come to consider the propagation of this impulse along the fiber in the direction of the arrow, we have to introduce the concept that, in addition to the ionic mechanisms of the surface membrane, the fiber as a whole is acting like a kind of cable. However, this cable property of the nerve is terribly poor by any engineering standards. In electrical transmission along a submarine cable there is a conducting core and an insulating sheath. In the nerve fiber the specific conductance of the core is about 10^8 times worse than the copper core that the electrical engineer would use. Moreover, the sheath is about 10^6 times leakier than that of a good cable. So the cable-like performance of a nerve fiber is about 10^8 × 10^6 times poorer. Nevertheless, in evolutionary design this very discouraging performance of the biological cable was circumvented by a device also used in cable transmissions over long distances, where attenuation becomes serious. Boosters are inserted at intervals to lift the attenuated signals.

In the nerve fiber a booster mechanism is built in all the way along the

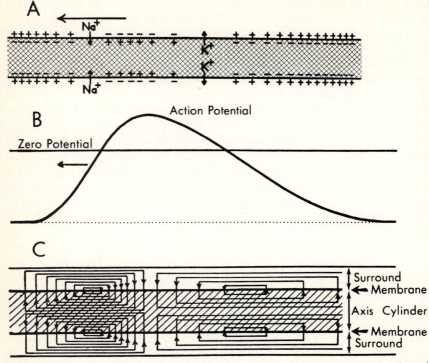

Figure 1-16 Ionic fluxes and current flow at an instant during the propagation of a nerve impulse. In *A* are the ionic fluxes, in *B* the membrane potential as in Fig. 1-15, and in *C* the lines of current flow between the axis cylinder and the surround, illustrating the cable properties of the nerve fiber. (*From Eccles, 1953.*)

surface. In Fig. 1-16*B* the impulse is drawn as if frozen in its propagation along the fiber, from right to left. It is shown in *C* that ahead of the impulse there is a passive cable-like spread with current leaving the outer surface of the fiber and circling back towards the impulse zone. Thus charge is taken off the membrane by this quite limited cable-like spread ahead of the impulse with the result that this zone becomes depolarized sufficiently to open the sodium gates (of Fig. 1-15) and so to turn on the self-regenerative process of sodium conductance that leads on to the full-sized potential change of the impulse. All that the cable-like property of the nerve fiber has to do is to transmit the depolarization for a minute distance along the surface. Then the booster mechanism of the membrane, i.e., the self-regenerative sodium conductance, takes over and builds the full impulse. The process goes on seriatim giving the indefinite propagation of a full-sized impulse.

Figure 1-16 thus gives in diagrammatic form the essential features of the ionic mechanism of nerve transmission that occurs for invertebrates and vertebrates. It is the explanation of the universal currency of the nervous system, and I think it is the most efficient biological mechanism that could have been developed for the fast transmission of messages over the relatively long distances required in large animals.

I have now explained how the impulse has moved along the fiber and how recovery occurs in its wake. The whole process has been accomplished with the loss of some potassium and the gain of some sodium. This ionic exchange has been measured by radiotracer techniques and is in good agreement with prediction. There is thus the further requirement that ionic recovery has to be brought about by ionic pumps such as those diagrammed in Fig. 1-13C. It has been found that the more sodium there is inside the stronger the pumps work, so there is an automatic recovery mechanism. But there is no urgency in this ionic restoration because nerve fibers contain enormously more ions than they need for one impulse. A squid giant axon only loses about one-millionth of its potassium per impulse, but the thinnest nerve fibers, with a much larger surface/volume ratio, may lose as much as one-thousandth. Nevertheless, there is an ionic reserve for hundreds of impulses, and meanwhile the ionic composition is continuously being restored by metabolically operated ionic pumps.

Figure 1-16C illustrates a remarkable property of impulse transmission. The cable-like spread ahead of the impulse is accomplished by electric currents that flow outwards from the membrane and thence through the surrounding medium to enter the membrane at the zone of the impulse and so to complete the circuit by return up the conducting core of the nerve fiber. In accord with predictions, alterations in the conductivity of the "surround" change the effectiveness of the cable-like spread, the conduction velocity being faster with increase and slower with decrease. It might be thought that this use of the surround for return current flow was an undesirable feature of design because an impulse on one fiber might spread to adjacent fibers (cross-talk) under the usual conditions of close packing. However, reference to Fig. 1-16C shows that the privacy of the fibers is safeguarded by virtue of the directions of current flow into adjacent fibers of the surround. Into them there is an initial strong anodal current before the cathodal current associated with the peak of action potential, and finally there is a terminal anodal current. As an impulse travels along a nerve fiber, adjacent fibers are subjected to the depressant action of anodal current before and after the cathodal current. Thus it is explained that cross-talk does not occur even with the closest packing of normal nerve fibers. However, injured regions of nerve fibers can be zones of cross-talk and this can result in sensory disturbances, as in causalgia and neuralgia.

It has long been known that a nerve impulse is followed by a period during which it is impossible to set up a second impulse (the absolutely refractory period) and the further period during which a stronger stimulus is required to set up an impulse (the relatively refractory period), which in addition is smaller in size. The usual illustrations from the older literature give a confused picture because they are recorded from nerve trunks often containing thousands of fibers. In contrast, Fig. 1-17 is an intracellular recording from a motor nerve fiber in a cat spinal cord of action potentials evoked by double stimulation of that fiber after it has left the spinal cord (cf. Fig. 1-6A). At B, with the shortest stimulus interval (0.7 ms), the second stimulus was ineffective, at C (0.8 ms) it was sometimes effective, the second action potential being depressed. As the stimulus interval was lengthened to 2.3 ms, D to E to F, the action potential recovered almost to full size.

This rapid recovery is typical of the nerve fibers in the brain. As a consequence nerve fibers can carry high frequencies of discharge. In Fig. 1-8B the highest frequencies of the motoneuronal discharge were over 200 per second. Discharge frequencies also exceeded 200 per second in Fig. 3-4A and 3-4B. But more remarkable are the extremely high frequencies

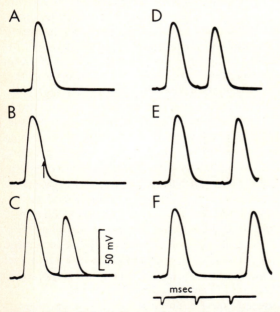

Figure 1-17 Refractoriness of nerve fiber. Intracellular recording from a motor axon in the cat spinal cord that was stimulated about 20 mm away, there being double stimulation in B to F. [J. S. Coombs, D. R. Curtis, and J. C. Eccles, J. Physiol., **139**:198 (1957).]

often attained by the discharges of many species of interneurons in the central nervous system. For example, in Fig. 3-9B the frequency of the Renshaw cell discharge was initially at 1600 per second; yet its axon carried this high frequency of impulses, though with a diminished size, and its synapses operated effectively for each successive impulse (Fig. 3-9C). Usually the absolutely refractory period for mammalian nerve fibers is about 0.5 ms. Evidently nerve fibers have a functional design that given a potentiality for frequency response adequate for the most extreme demands made by intensely discharging neurons.

CONDUCTION VELOCITY AND THE MYELINATED FIBERS

Now we come to a disadvantage that is inherent in the initial invertebrate design of the nerve fiber as a conducting device. The disadvantage is that the conduction velocity is slow. If the impulse is to glide along the fiber in the manner of successive invasion by the cable transmission and supplementary boosting as in Fig. 1-16, the progress is slow. For example, with a large crab axon 30 μm in diameter the conduction velocity is only 5 m/s. The cable transmission is more expeditious if the fiber diameter is larger, but, if other factors are unchanged, it can be shown theoretically that the reward in speed is disappointing, for it is proportional to the square root of the diameter. Thus, in accordance with expectation, increasing the diameter by 16 times, as from crab axon to squid axon (30 μm to 500 μm), gives only a fourfold increase in velocity, i.e., from 5 to 20 m/s.

   And so the invertebrates such as the squid were caught in a dilemma. As they developed in size and needed to retain their quickness of response, progressively more of their bulk had to be devoted to nerve fibers. For example, a doubling of bodily dimensions would entail an increase of 4-fold in diameter and 16-fold in cross-sectional area of nerve fibers to give the same conduction time for a doubling of conduction distance. Thus, for a linear doubling of dimensions, the mass of the animal would go up 8 times and the bulk of a nerve fiber by 32 times. Evidently the squid has gone about as far as evolutionarily possible with the development of such giant nerve fibers, in order to effect a contraction of the mantle musculature, its escape mechanism, with maximum expedition. And all the squid can afford is one of these giant fibers in each mantle nerve (Fig. 1-10B) with the consequence that it has an all-or-nothing movement with no gradation.

   The situation was transformed by the brilliant innovation of coating the nerve fibers by a thick insulation that was interrupted at intervals. Actually this innovation was foreshadowed by an invertebrate, the prawn, that achieved the velocity of the squid giant axon with a fiber diameter of only 20 μm. But the vertebrates perfected the design. Figure 1-18*B* illustrates the essential features of impulse conduction in a nerve fiber coated by the insulating myelin sheath, in contrast to the unmyelinated fiber in Fig. 1-18*A*. In Fig. 1-18*A* the impulse glides along the fiber by smooth progressive cable invasion as in Fig. 1-16. In Fig. 1-18*B* only the spaced nodal interruptions of the myelin sheath are active in the propagation, and the cable transmission is by currents flowing from the inactive node at the left into the active node with its reverse membrane potential. There is thus activation in succession of node to node without any active contribution from the long internodal zones. Actually the myelinated fiber in Fig. 1-18*B* is drawn distorted by the large transverse magnification shown by the scale. In the undistorted drawing of Fig. 1-18*C* the relative lengths of nodes and internodes can be appreciated for an ordinary large vertebrate nerve fiber.

Extraordinary efficiency is achieved by the design of having the impulse hop from node to node (the so-called *saltatory transmission*) with the long internodal section passive. It is often mistakenly thought that the myelin sheath achieves this remarkable result simply because it is an insulator preventing the flow of current across the nerve membrane of the internode. However at least as important a contribution by the myelin sheath is given by the enormous reduction (to less than 1 percent) in the electrical capacity between the axis cylinder and the surround. This reduction simply results from the increased plate separation of the

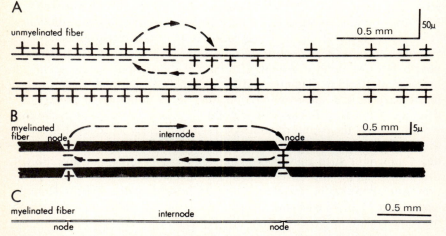

Figure 1-18 Propagation of impulse along a nerve fiber. In *A* there is propagation as in Fig. 1-16*C*, but with only one line of current flow drawn in. In *B* the propagation is in a myelinated fiber, with the current flow restricted to the nodes. The dimensions in *B* are transversely exaggerated as shown by the scale, but are correctly shown in *C*. (*Modified from Hodgkin, 1964.*)

cylindrical condenser enveloping the fiber in the internodes. It is for this reason that the brief currents shown in Fig. 1-18*B* spread so effectively from node to node even with the long distances shown in Fig. 1-18*C*. No more than half of the inward current at an active node is lost by leakage through the resistance and capacity of the myelinated membrane of the internode.

Figure 1-19*A* shows diagrammatically the myelin wrapping around the internode and the manner of its interruption at the node, where the bare nerve membrane has channels for Na^+ and K^+ ions controlled by gates, just as for the surface of an unmyelinated fiber (Fig. 1-15), but at a considerably greater density. Since the booster operations by ionic fluxes during activity are restricted to less than 1 percent of the surface area of the nerve fiber, the ionic fluxes are greatly reduced. Hence, there is an enormous metabolic advantage in myelination.

Figure 1-19*B*, *C*, and *D* illustrates the remarkable manner in which the spiral wrapping of myelin is applied to the nerve fiber. There is one enveloping cell called a *Schwann cell* around each internode (*B*). Then it

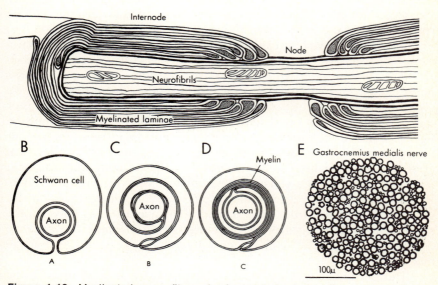

Figure 1-19 Myelinated nerve fibers. In *A* a node is shown diagrammatically in a longitudinal section. The terminals of the laminated myelin wrapping are shown applied to the surface of the nerve fiber adjacent to the node. Also shown are the neurofibrils and three mitochondria. *B*, *C*, and *D* show sequences in the formation of the myelin sheath by the rotatory migration of the Schwann cell. [*J. D. Robertson, J. Biophys. Biochem Cytol.*, **4:**349 (1958).] *E* shows the tight packing of myelinated fibers of a wide range in size in a muscle nerve of the cat. [*J. C. Eccles and C. S. Sherrington, Proc. Roy. Soc. B*, **106:**326 (1930).]

starts a spiral migration around the fiber, wrapping its surface membrane around in layer after layer. All the Schwann cell cytoplasm is eventually squeezed out as the wrapping continues (C and D) so that there is left just the myelin sheath, with layer after layer of two opposed Schwann cell membranes, each of about 85-Å thickness. In a large nerve fiber there may be more than 100 of the double membranes. Thus the myelin wrapping of each internode is the creation of a single Schwann cell. It is remarkable that with respect to the direction of the spiral wrapping there is no collusion between Schwann cells of adjacent internodes.

Figure 1-19E is a transverse section of a mammalian nerve, showing the dark myelin sheath around the fibers, the wide variation in fiber size and the close packing of the fibers. Yet, as we have seen, though its transmission is by electric currents, there is no risk of cross-talk. The conduction velocity is approximately proportional to the fiber diameter, the ratio being about 6:1 for mammalian nerves. Thus a large nerve fiber of 20 μm in diameter (including the myelin) would conduct impulses at about 120 m/s. It should be mentioned that all large nerve fibers in the brain also have a myelin sheath. Impulse conduction is comparable with that in peripheral nerve. The only difference is that the myelin is made by the oligodendroglia, which are a special variety of glial cells that will be referred to at the end of Chap. 5.

Figure 1-20 gives an elegant demonstration of the way in which a nerve impulse hops from node to node, as was first discovered by Tasaki and then fully investigated by Huxley and Stämpfli. Diagram B shows a nerve fiber with two nodes in a rat dorsal rootlet. Recording is by two electrodes on the nerve fiber at the positions indicated by the two stems of the "Y," about 350 μm apart, and these are moved progressively along the fiber as shown. The impulse propagates downwards (arrow). In the four upper records of A there is no change in the time of the electrical response until the brief delay as the electrodes record from the next internode, then again a constant time until crossing the third internode. Plotting of the latency against distance (Fig. 1-20C) shows this stepwise delay in the impulse from node to node. The average time between the successive nodal invasions is very brief (25 μs). Since the distance between nodes was 1.25 mm, the conduction velocity would be about 50 m/s.

This technique is very valuable in disclosing local defects in the myelin sheath. They can be produced experimentally by diphtheria toxin. With mild damage there is delay at each node so that the internodal time may increase from 25 μs to as long as 300 μs under conditions just critical for blockage. This diphtheria damage provides an experimental model for the state of the nerve fibers in the pathways to and from the brain in the disease called *multiple sclerosis*. For an as yet unknown reason the myelin of the nerve fibers disintegrates, hence the failure of impulse transmission

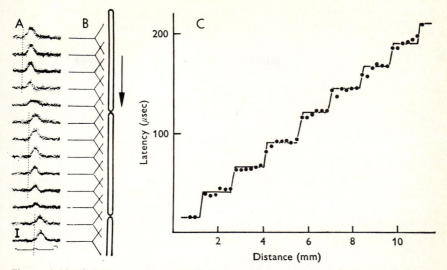

Figure 1-20 Saltatory conduction along a myelinated fiber. The fiber is shown in *B* with two nodes, the arrow giving the direction of propagation. The fiber is in a very fine filament of a spinal cord root and recordings of the impulse are made by two fine electrodes about 350 μm apart that are applied as shown at various positions along the nerve fiber. Note in *B* the two forks of the Y's whose stems point to the recorded potentials in *A*. In *A* the vertical dotted lines define three sets of records with simultaneous onsets and with steps of 25 μs between. In *C* are plotted measurements showing eight steps in another fiber. [*M. Rasminsky and T. A. Sears, J. Physiol., 217:66P (1971).*]

and the resultant severe incapacity. The nerve fibers are not killed, so there is hope that the disease could be cured if they can have their myelin wrapping restored. The prospects for success are much brighter than for diseases where the nerve cells and fibers have died.

A remarkable feature of mammalian nerves is the extremely wide range of fiber diameters (cf. Fig. 1-19*E*). This wide variation also occurs in the brain and in the pathways to and from the brain. This finding has to be considered in relation to impulse conduction velocity, the velocity in meters per second being approximately equal to six times the diameter in microns. Thus the range in velocities for the normal range of myelinated fiber diameter, 2 to 20 μm, would be 12 to 120 m/s. In addition there are extremely numerous unmyelinated fibers from 0.2 to 1.0 μm in diameter that have much slower velocities—0.2 to 2 m/s. There is much evidence for the attractive postulate that the fiber velocity is related to the urgency of the information it is called upon to transmit. The fastest fibers are concerned in the control of movement, both the afferent input from muscles (cf. Fig. 1-8*A*) and so up to the brain and the descending pathways from the brain to muscles. Some of the pathways of cutaneous sense (cf. Fig. 1-7A) are also fast. At the other extreme, pathways carrying visceral information are not urgent and are slowly conducting; they are even unmyelinated over much of their course. In general it can be postulated that, in the evolutionary design of the nervous system, nerve fiber size is related to the urgency of the information it carries. More simply put: nerve fibers are no larger than they should be!

REFERENCES

Akert, K., H. Moor, K. Pfenninger, and C. Sandri (1968): "Contributions of New Impregnation Methods and Freeze Etching to the Problems of Synaptic Fine Structure," in K. Akert and P. G. Waser (eds.), *Progress in Brain Research*, vol. 31, *Mechanisms of Synaptic Transmission*, Elsevier, Amsterdam, pp. 223–240.

Akert, K., K. Peper, and C. Sandri (1975): "Structural Organization of Motor End Plate and Central Synapses," in P. G. Waser (ed.), *Cholinergic Mechanisms*, Raven Press, New York, pp. 43–57.

Bezanilla, F., and C. M. Armstrong (1975): "Kinetic Properties and Inactivation of Gating Currents of Sodium Channels in Squid Axon," *Phil. Trans. R. Soc. Lond. B.*, **270**:449–458.

Conradi, S. (1969): "Ultrastructure of Dorsal Root Boutons on Lumbosacral Motoneurons of the Adult Cat, as Revealed by Dorsal Root Section," *Acta Physiol., Scand. Suppl.*, **332**:85–115.

De Robertis, E. (1971): "Molecular Biology of Synaptic Receptors," *Science*, **171**:963–971.

De Robertis, E. (1975): *Synaptic Receptors, Isolation and Molecular Biology*, Marcel Dekker, New York, p. 387.

Fox, C. F. (1972): "The Structure of Cell Membranes," *Sci. Amer.*, **226**:31–38.

Gray, E. G. (1969): "Electron Microscopy of Excitatory and Inhibitory Synapses: A Brief Review," in K. Akert and P. G. Waser (eds.), *Progress in Brain Research*, vol. 31, *Mechanisms of Synaptic Transmission*, Elsevier, Amsterdam, pp. 141–155.

Gray, E. G. (1970): "The Fine Structure of Nerve," *Comp. Biochem. Physiol.*, **36**:419–448.

Hodgkin, A. L. (1958): "Ionic Movements and Electrical Activity in Giant Nerve Fibres," *Proc. Roy Soc. B*, **148**:1–37.

Hodgkin, A. L. (1964): *The Conduction of the Nervous Impulse*, Liverpool University Press, Liverpool.

Huxley, A. F. (1959): "Ion Movements during Nerve Activity," *Ann N.Y. Acad. Sci.*, **81**:221–246.

Huxley, A. F., and R. Stämpfli (1949): "Evidence for Saltatory Conduction in Peripheral Myelinated Nerve Fibres," *J. Physiol.*, **108**:315–339.

Katz, B. (1966): *Nerve, Muscle, and Synapse*, McGraw-Hill, New York.

Keynes, R. D. (1958): "The Nerve Impulse and the Squid," *Sci. Amer.*, 1958; reprinted in *Physiological Psychology*, Freeman, San Francisco, 1971, pp. 128–135.

Mountcastle, V. B. (1966): "The Neural Replication of Sensory Events in the Somatic Afferent System," in J. C. Eccles (ed.), *Brain and Conscious Experience*, Springer, New York, pp. 85–115.

Mountcastle, V. B. (1975): "The View from Within: Pathways to the Study of Perception," *The Johns Hopkins Medical Journal*, **136:**109–131.

Reisfeld, R. A., and B. D. Kahan (1972): "Markers of Biological Individuality," *Sci. Amer.*, **226:**28–37.

Rojas, E. and R. D. Keynes (1975): "On the Relation Between Displacement Currents and Activation of the Sodium Conductances in the Squid Giant Axon," *Phil. Trans. R. Soc. Lond. B.*, **270:**459–482.

Peripheral
Synaptic Transmission

Before embarking on the attempt to study neuronal mechanisms in the brain, it is important to study the transmission at peripheral synapses because the investigations on some of these synapses provide the basis for our understanding of synapses in the brain. Essentially the same biological processes go on in the central synapses in the brain, but they are more elusive when it comes to such precise investigations as I am going to discuss in this chapter. Of the many peripheral synapses that have been studied, I choose the three in which the highest scientific standards have been attained: neuromuscular synapses, especially in the frog and snake; the giant synapses in the stellate ganglion of the squid; and the synapses on the ganglion cells in the frog heart. These three exemplars of peripheral synapses form an adequate experimental base for the understanding of the essential features of central synapses. Their scientific investigation will be described in Chap. 3.

NEUROMUSCULAR TRANSMISSION

Introduction

Figure 2-1 is a diagram that serves to introduce the subject. The motoneuron has already been described in the preceding chapter. From the motoneuron there projects the myelinated axon, a nerve fiber, that extends all the way down to muscle. This myelinated axon has nodes, so an impulse discharged from the motoneuron (and that is the story of the next chapter) hops from node to node down to the muscle with a speed of propagation of about 80 m/s (see Fig. 1-20). Thus a motoneuronal discharge quickly results in a muscle response even when the distance is 1 m, as it is from motoneurons in our spinal cord to our foot muscles. The nerve fiber then branches and the impulse traverses all the branches at full size because it is an all-or-nothing process with a good safety factor in its propagation. Usually in the propagation of a nerve impulse there is a safety factor of about five, so it can invade all the branches of a fairly profuse terminal arborization.

In Fig. 2-1 there are branches only to five muscle fibers, each with a little terminal efflorescence of the nerve fiber. Our problem concerns what is happening when the impulse travels to the end of these terminals on the muscle fibers. How does it cause an impulse discharge along each of the muscle fibers, which is a prerequisite for the muscle contraction? (It should be noted that the correct number of terminal branches is much more than shown. Usually it is 100 to 200.) Furthermore, any muscle fiber as a rule (there are exceptions, but they are rare) has only one nerve fiber innervating it, and the impulse propagation from nerve to muscle has a good safety factor, also usually of about five, so that it doesn't break down under any biological conditions. Thus this nerve cell can fire impulses at any of the frequencies of its normal operation, as for example in Fig. 1-8B, and be sure that the requisite muscle contraction will ensue. All movements, every action you have ever carried out is a result of this transmission from motoneuron discharge to muscle contraction. There is no other way in which a body can perform any action that requires its musculature.

Figure 2-1C shows that, within limits, the higher the frequency of the nerve cell discharge, the larger the resulting contraction. There are three rather separate twitches of the muscle when the frequency of discharge from the single motoneuron is 10 per second. At 20 per second the contraction tends to fuse and this tendency increases at 32 and at 50, until at 80 per second there is a smooth, strong contraction. It is perhaps somewhat surprising that a single cat motoneuron can command a contraction of 100 grams (g) in one of the leg muscles. In man the unit contraction would be higher, but it is not accurately known. Thus stronger

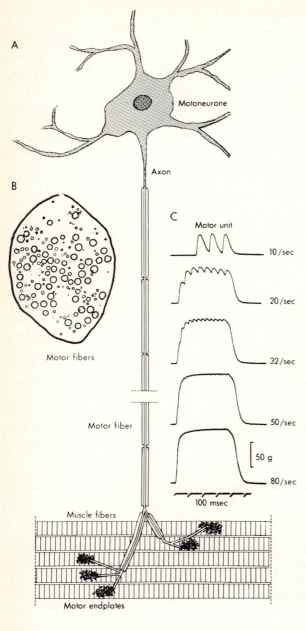

Figure 2-1 The motor unit. *A.* Motoneuron with its axon passing as a myelinated nerve fiber to innervate muscle fibers. *B.* Transverse section of motor fibers supplying a cat muscle, all afferent fibers having degenerated. [*J. C. Eccles and C. S. Sherrington, Proc. Roy. Soc. B, 106:326 (1930).*] *C.* Isometric mechanical responses of a single motor unit of the cat gastrocnemius muscle. The responses were evoked by repetitive stimulation of the motoneuron (cf. *A*) by pulses of current applied through an intracellular electrode at the indicated frequencies in cycles per second. [*M. S. Devanandan, R. M. Eccles, and R. A. Westerman, J. Physiol., 178:359 (1965).*]

actions of your muscles are secured by faster firing of your motoneurons. But more effective is the bringing into action of many more motoneurons. Any large muscle has many hundreds of motoneurons innervating it. In

Fig. 2-1*B* there are about 60 large motor axons in the transverse section (cf. Fig. 1-19*E*) of a nerve branch to a cat muscle.

This introduces us to the concept of the *motor unit*, which may be defined as the motor nerve fiber and all the muscle fibers innervated by it. This concept was developed by Sherrington. He, for the first time, arrived at the correct idea that all movements are ensembles or composites of contractions of individual motor units. Various fractions of the total number are excited, depending on the strength of contraction that is needed for any particular action, i.e., the total motoneuron pool of the muscle with its motoneurons is fractionated from moment to moment according to needs. And the total number of motoneurons with their dependent motor units is about 200,000 for the human spinal cord. That number is responsible for the contractions of all the muscles of the limbs, body, and neck, i.e., for our total muscular performance except for the head. It is remarkable that we can learn to activate individual motoneurons in arm or leg muscles, and to switch now to one, now to another at will. This has been demonstrated in elegant experiments by Basmajian in which the distinctive electrical responses of several contracting motor units of a muscle were displayed on the screen of a cathode-ray oscilloscope, and the subject could learn voluntarily to "play" one or the other.

The transmission from a nerve impulse to a muscle impulse is the first example of chemical synaptic transmission that was securely established. For a long time many investigators thought that the transmission time of one-thousandth of a second was too fast for chemical mediation. Thirty or forty years ago there was the alternative postulate that the electric currents of the nerve impulse directly excited the muscle fiber. Many synapses are now known where this electrical transmission does occur, but, because of the large electrical mismatch between the tiny nerve fiber and the large muscle fiber, electrical transmission is ineffective by at least two orders of magnitude. Transmission is entirely due to chemical mediation by a substance called *acetylcholine* (ACh), as was originally proposed by Dale and his colleagues in the 1930s. Earlier still, in the 1920s, Loewi had established that chemical transmission is responsible for the vagal inhibition of the heart, and this transmitter also was eventually shown to be ACh. In 1936 Loewi and Dale were jointly awarded Nobel prizes for their discoveries.

Structural Features of the Neuromuscular Synapse
In the mammal the nerve terminal is a tightly clustered structure on the surface of the muscle fiber, as indicated in Fig. 2-1*A* and as drawn in microscopic section in Fig. 2-2*A*, where the axon (ax) makes three small contacts on the surface of the muscle fiber (mf) but doesn't fuse with it. There is the separation that is characteristic of all chemical synapses and

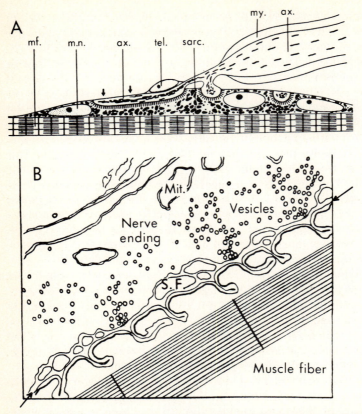

Figure 2-2 Microscopic structure of neuromuscular synapses. *A.* Schematic drawing of a motor endplate: ax., axoplasm with its mitochondria; my., myelin sheath; tel., teloglia (terminal Schwann cells); sarc., sarcoplasm of muscle fiber with its mitochondria; m.n., muscle nuclei; mf., muscle fiber. The terminal nerve branches lie in "troughs." [*R. Couteaux, Exp. Cell. Res. Suppl., 5:294 (1958).*] *B.* Drawing of electron micrograph of part of neuromuscular junction from frog sartorius. Longitudinal section of the muscle. [*R. Birks, H. E. Huxley, and B. Katz, J. Physiol., 150:134 (1960).*]

that has been displayed in brain synapses in Figs. 1-3, 1-4, and 1-5. The special structural enlargement of the sarcoplasm (sarc) of the muscle fiber at the junctional region is called a *motor endplate*. The problem is that the nerve impulse travels down to the nerve ending and after only one-thousandth of a second of transmission time a new impulse starts up in the muscle fiber at the region of the endplate and runs along it in both directions, so setting up the contraction.

However, light microscopy, good as it was, was not adequate to reveal the essential structures of the nerve-muscle synapse. It was only with the advent of electron microscopy that the structural bases of chemical transmission were revealed. The frog neuromuscular synapse is much less compact than that in the mammal. Fine nerve fibers run for hundreds of microns in longitudinal grooves on the surface of the muscle fiber, as is well illustrated in the drawings from a microphotograph in Fig. 2-4, where two such fibers are shown. In Fig. 2-2*B* there is a drawing showing an electron micrograph of a longitudinal section of a segment of one such long nerve fiber in the frog. The muscle can be recognized by the longidutinal striations with two transverse striations. The nerve terminal can be recognized by the dense aggregation of vesicles, with mitochondria (Mit.) lying further back from the muscle. The surface of the muscle fiber is shown by the dense line with frequent foldings. Opposite three of the foldings are clusters of synaptic vesicles, but in several places small projections, S.F., from the enveloping Schwann cell intrude between the nerve and muscle surfaces. Elsewhere there is separation by a cleft of about 400 Å across, as marked by the arrow on each side. The numerous spherical vesicles are about 500 Å in diameter and are characteristic of all chemically transmitting synapses (cf. Figs. 1-3*B*, 1-4*B*, and 1-5); hence, they are appropriately called *synaptic vesicles.*

There are two essential structural features of a chemical synapse, as is illustrated in Fig. 1-5—first the synaptic vesicles and then the *synaptic cleft,* the space (note arrows in Fig. 2-2) across which transmission has to occur. As illustrated in Fig. 3-3*A* and *B*, this synaptic cleft provides the essential space for currents to flow that are generated by the action of the transmitter substance on the membrane across the synapse—the *postsynaptic membrane*— in this case the membrane of the motor endplate.

The essential mechanism of the synapse is that the nerve impulse causes some of the synaptic vesicles to liberate their contents into the synaptic cleft. These vesicles contain prepackaged acetylcholine, about 5000 molecules of acetylcholine in each according to latest estimates (see below); and they squirt their contents into the synaptic cleft. By diffusion across the cleft the acetylcholine acts on the membrane of the motor endplate which is folded in order to increase its area. The transmitter opens the ionic gates and ions stream through, causing a change in membrane potential of the muscle fiber in the direction of a depolarization. When this reaches a critical level, a muscle impulse is generated that propagates along the muscle fiber and sets off the complex sequence of events responsible for a muscle contraction. We now turn to consider in some detail the experiments by which this synaptic mechanism has been revealed. Special reference should be made to two books by Katz: *Nerve, Muscle, and Synapse* and *The Release of Neural Transmitter Substances.*

Physiological Features of the Neuromuscular Synapse

I am attempting to give the essential physiology, not a detailed biophysical account, but sufficient for understanding the synaptic mechanisms in the brain, which will be the theme of the next chapter. In Fig. 2-3*A* there is

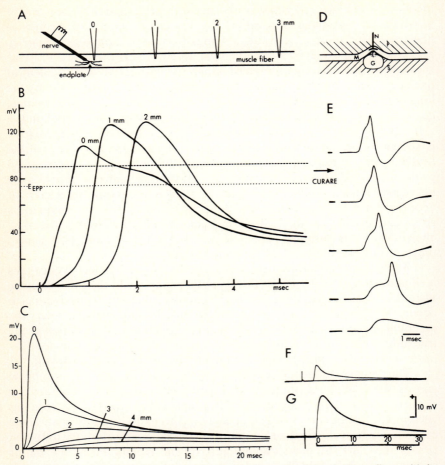

Figure 2-3 Endplate potentials and muscle action potentials. *A.* Nerve fiber with its terminal branches innervating a frog muscle fiber. *B.* Action potentials evoked by a single nerve impulse and recorded as in *A* at 0, 1, and 2 mm from the motor endplate. The broken line gives the level of zero membrane potential, the resting membrane potential being −90 mV. The dotted line is at the equilibrium potential for the endplate potential (E_{EPP}). *C.* Action potentials evoked and recorded as in *B*, but after blockage of neuromuscular transmission by curare. [*P. Fatt and B. Katz, J. Physiol.*, **115**:320 (1951).] *D.* Isolated single nerve (N)-muscle (M) preparation that was mounted on a recording electrode. *E.* Series of potentials recorded as in *D* showing progressive action of curare. [*S. W. Kuffler, J. Neurophysiol.*, **5**:18 (1942).] *F,G.* EPPs of curarized muscle recorded at endplate region as in *C* before and after addition of 10^{-6} prostigmine. [*P. Fatt and B. Katz, J. Physiol.*, **115**:320 (1951).]

a nerve fiber terminating on the motor endplate, with the fine nerve terminals running along the muscle fiber as in Fig. 2-4*A*. We can stimulate the nerve fiber by a brief electrical pulse through the applied electrode and so send an impulse down to the nerve terminal as described in Chap. 1. Recording from the muscle fiber is, as shown in Fig. 2-3A, by an intracellular microelectrode either right at the motor endplate or at 1, 2, or 3 mm away.

At all sites the potential across the muscle membrane is about 90 mV, inside negative, which is the normal value for a frog muscle fiber. Just as with the giant nerve fiber in Fig. 1-11, when the microelectrode crosses the membrane, there is immediately registered a membrane potential of -90 mV. In Fig. 2-3B with recording at the motor endplate (0 mm), a nerve impulse evoked, after a brief latency, a complex potential change with humps on the rising and falling phases that will be explained later. At 1 and 2 mm away the response looks simpler. It rises rapidly and smoothly, and starts to go down just like an ordinary nerve impulse (Figs. 1-14 and 1-17), but it is greatly slowed in its latter part. Two changes have occurred in moving away from the motor endplate. One is that the impulse is later. That is because the muscle impulse started at the endplate and moved along, just as with an impulse in a nerve fiber except that it is much slower, only about 1 m/s. The other is that the humps have disappeared, and the summit is higher. How can this be explained? What is happening at the endplate zone that reduces the muscle action potential and adds the humps before and after? The answer is that a special operation due to the chemical transmitter effects these changes at the endplate.

The initial hump is in fact due to depolarization by the transmitter, and at a critical level of this depolarization (about 50 mV), it can be seen to fire the impulse. But this impulse is much smaller than at 1 or 2 mm from the endplate. Evidently the transmitter action on the endplate membrane is preventing the impulse from reaching as high a reversal point as elsewhere. The transmitter depolarization has an equilibrium potential (E_{EPP}) at about -15 mV (dotted line), so effectively it pulls the muscle impulse potential down toward this value. The ionic mechanism of the impulse would tend to give a membrane potential of at least $+40$ mV, just as has been seen with the nerve impulse in Figs. 1-14 and 1-16. The net result is the compromise at about $+15$ mV for the summit of the action potential at the endplate (0 mm). Finally the depolarization by the residual transmitter action satisfactorily explains the hump on the declining phase of the impulse at the endplate. These endplate effects are very slight at 1 mm and virtually absent at 2 mm.

If the size of the endplate potential could be reduced so that it failed to fire an impulse, it would be much simpler to investigate the events at the neuromuscular synapse. This can be done by poisoning with curare. Curare was used for this purpose by the South American Indians as an arrow poison. They tipped their arrows with this plant extract and so paralyzed their enemies—an early example of chemical or biological warfare! In recent years curare or related substances have become clinically of great value because the anesthetist can in this way greatly depress neuromuscular transmission so that the surgeon can operate with the advantage of having the patient with perfect muscular relaxation.

Figure 2-3*D* and *E* gives a good illustration of progressive curarization. In the early 1940s, about 10 years before intracellular recording, Kuffler dissected out a single nerve-muscle fiber, seen in Fig. 2-3*D* (N,M), and could hold it between paraffin (P) and saline (S) while recording by a fine platinum wire supported by a curved glass rod, shown in transverse section in G. It was the first example of an investigation on a single nerve-muscle preparation in isolation. When the nerve is stimulated and the recording is from the endplate zone, E, there is a local potential followed by an action potential just as in Fig. 2-3*B*. After curare is added to the saline there is a progressive change, as is shown in the subsequent records of E. The initial potential was progressively reduced and fired the impulse progressively later, eventually failing. The muscle is now paralyzed. Until that happened the muscle action potential was full-sized. It is a beautiful example of the all-or-nothing. The nerve impulse either fires a full-sized muscle action potential or it doesn't fire.

As will be described below, curare works simply by preventing the acetylcholine from effectively depolarizing the muscle at the endplate. When the muscle impulse fails, there remains the *endplate potential* (EPP), as in the lowest trace of Fig. 2-3*E*. In Fig. 2-3*C* there are superimposed traces of such endplate potentials recorded intracellularly as in Fig. 2-3*A* at the endplate zone (0) and at 1, 2, 3, and 4 mm distal thereto. The endplate potential is decremented progressively with distances and becomes slower in time course. It is spreading simply by the cable properties of the muscle fiber, approximately halving every millimeter, so it becomes very much depleted from 0 to 1 to 2 to 3 to 4 mm. Cable transmission is even poorer in muscle fibers than in nerve fibers.

Pharmacological Properties of the Neuromuscular Synapse

We now can ask the question: How was it established that the transmitter is acetylcholine? Firstly, Dale and his colleagues showed very early that, when the nerve to a big muscle was stimulated and the venous effluent collected, acetylcholine was liberated into the effluent during a severe tetanization. Secondly, they showed that intra-arterial injection of acetylcholine caused the generation of impulse discharges in muscles with the associated contraction. Thirdly, substances (anticholinesterases) that prevented the enzymatic destruction of acetylcholine converted the neurally evoked response of the muscle from a single twitch to a brief waning tetanus, as would be expected if the transmission was due to a jet of acetylcholine. Though this work seems pretty crude by present standards, it was a remarkable achievement at that time.

A great improvement came with the electrophoretic injection of acetylcholine out of a fine micropipette that could be manipulated into very close proximity to a motor endplate. Recording was by an intracellular electrode in a preparation that was curarized so that only an endplate potential was evoked, much as in Fig. 2-3C at 0. With the best location, Krnjevic and Miledi found that electrophoretic injection of 1.5×10^{-14} g of acetylcholine just outside the muscle endplate gave a potential very similar to that produced by a nerve impulse that is estimated to liberate 1.5×10^{-15} g at the endplate. This discrepancy by a factor of 10 is as good as can be expected when it is remembered that the injection could only be at one side of the cleft, whereas the acetylcholine liberated by the nerve impulse would be directly onto the endplate surface (cf. Fig. 2-2) and would be acting over the whole of this surface.

A still higher level of technical excellence has been achieved recently by McMahan, Kuffler, and their associates. In Fig. 2-4A the drawing is from a photomicrograph of a living muscle fiber identified by its cross striations, and on its surface can be seen two terminal nerve fibers running longitudinally. This beautiful display is due to a special technique called Nomarski interference microscopy, which allows the living tissue to be studied with very high magnification, and with sharp optical sections. It is a particularly good arrangement for the experimenter to have the two nerve fibers so nicely parallel and terminating together. Below the graph (B) you can see the muscle fiber in section with the two nerve terminals in little grooves (a and d). The muscle fiber has a recording intracellular electrode that is out of the picture in A, but at a distance that is quite small, relative to the length constant of the muscle fiber, so that it would record with little distortion the potential changes across the muscle membrane.

Electrophoretic injections of acetylcholine were made by the micropipette, E, that is shown accurately applied at point (c) on the muscle membrane between the two nerve terminals. The injecting current was 3.2×10^{-8} A for 1 ms, and the applied points are shown as black dots along the line between the two nerve terminals. When the point of application (a in A) was close to the visualized nerve terminal, it produced in B and C the large depolarization labeled a. The same injection only about 5 μm away (b in A) gave the smaller depolarization (b), while, when injection was between the two nerve terminals (c in A), the acetylcholine was hardly affecting the membrane at all (c). Finally, when the injection was near (d in A) to the other nerve terminal, there was the large response (d) again. The results of several additional injections as well are plotted in the

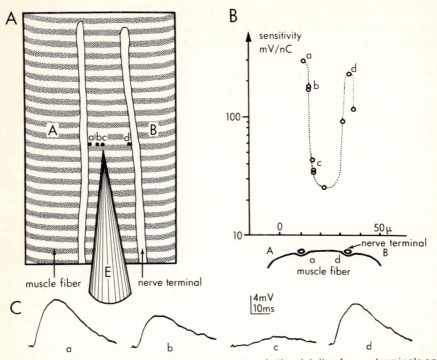

Figure 2-4 Distribution of acetylcholine receptors in the vicinity of nerve terminals on skeletal muscle of the frog. Full description in the text. (*From Pepper and McMahan, 1972.*)

graph and show how subtle and delicate this performance is, the two nerve terminals being shown below *B* on the same scale.

Now what does this show? It is showing most beautifully just this—that only the muscle membrane under the nerve fibers is sensitive to acetylcholine. The remainder is not sensitive at all. The apparent effects at other sites are due to diffusion of the injected acetycholine onto the sensitive sites at the nerve contacts. The same decrement of response, as from *a* to *c*, is observed if the tip of the electrode is moved vertically away from the nerve fiber area. It can be concluded that the sensitivity to acetylcholine is exactly at the actual groove, just where the nerve contact is.

A still more exquisite experiment has recently been carried out by Kuffler and associates on the synapses on snake muscle fibers. Pretreatment by collaginase to remove fibrous tissue allows the nerve terminal with the whole presynaptic apparatus to be gently lifted off the postsynaptic sites, which remain as "craters" directly accessible to the electrophoretic application of ACh (cf. Fig. 2-9D). High sensitivity to ACh is found to be restricted precisely to the "craters." Quantitative details follow after the next section.

The Quantal Liberation of Acetylcholine

We now come to an investigation relating the liberation of acetylcholine (ACh) to the vesicles that are seen in the nerve terminal in Fig. 2-2B. It is based largely on the classical experimental work of Katz, Fatt, Miledi, and their associates. In fact, at least two years before the vesicles had been recognized by electron microscopy there was evidence that the ACh was liberated from nerve terminals in packages.

In Fig. 2-5A the microelectrode was inserted into the muscle fiber quite close to the motor endplate. When in 1952 Fatt and Katz first detected the sequence of irregularly recurring small potentials, as shown in the upper traces of Fig. 2-5A, they did not realize at first that this "biological noise" was a major discovery. The accurate location of the recording electrode at the endplate is shown by the action potential with an initial EPP set up by a nerve impulse in the lowest trace of Fig. 2-5A, which resembles that in Fig. 2-3B at 0. When in Fig. 2-5B the recording electrode was 2 mm away, there was the simple action potential (cf. Fig. 2-3B) and almost no "biological noise," just traces attributable to cable transmission.

How can it be shown that this "biological noise" is due to acetylcholine? First, there is the action of curare which depresses the endplate potential and the "biological noise" in the same way. Figure 2-5C and D shows another test. An electrophoretic injection of ACh at the endplate region caused a brief depolarization as in Fig. 2-4. The lower traces of Fig. 2-5C show "biological noise" as in Fig. 2-5A, but at a much slower frequency. In Fig. 2-5D the electrophoretic injection of ACh is preceded by a substance edrophonium that very rapidly inactivates *acetylcholine esterase*, which is the enzyme that rapidly destroys ACh. Edrophonium works so rapidly that, when injected at E just before the ACh, the depolarization produced by the ACh jet was increased and prolonged because the ACh was not being destroyed by the acetylcholine esterase. At the same time in the lower traces of D it can be seen that the units of the biological noise were increased and prolonged. This is good evidence that the "biological noise" is due to brief jets of ACh that are acting on the endplate membrane of the muscle fiber. In every respect these miniature potentials have the properties of the endplate potential (EPP); hence, the justification of their designation as *miniature endplate potentials (min. EPP)*.

As soon as synaptic vesicles were discovered in electron micrographs of the nerve terminals (Fig. 2-2B), it was an attractive hypothesis

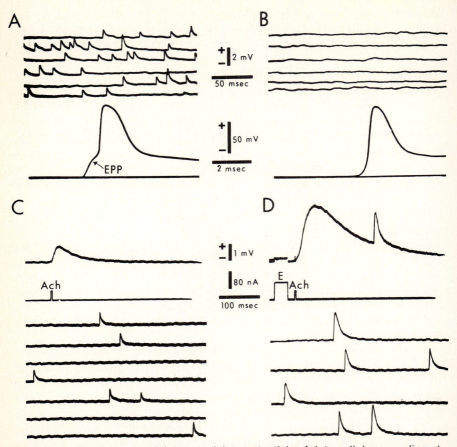

Figure 2-5 Spontaneous miniature endplate potentials. *A.* Intracellular recording at an endplate. *B.* Recorded 2 mm away in the same muscle fiber. Upper portions were recorded at low speed and high amplification: they show the localized spontaneous activity at the endplate region. Lower records show the electrical response to a nerve impulse, taken at high speed and lower gain (cf. Fig. 2-3*B*). [*P. Fatt and B. Katz, J. Physiol., 117:109 (1952).*] *C,D.* Upper traces show the potentiating effect of edrophonium (applied by pulse E) on endplate depolarization produced by a brief pulse of acetylcholine (ACh). In lower traces it is seen that the spontaneous miniature EPPs in *C* are greatly increased and prolonged in *D* during steady electrophoretic application of edrophonium. (*From Katz, 1969.*)

that they were packages of ACh and that these *quanta* were being liberated spontaneously in a random manner from the nerve terminal, so generating the miniature EPPs. Yet it has been fashionable to doubt this identification. My own comment was the reverse. I used to say that, if electron microscopy had not revealed the existence in nerve terminals of vesicles with properties appropriate for prepackaged transmitter, the prepackaging of transmitter would still have to be postulated, with the additional proviso that for some reason you couldn't see the packages! But now with electron microscopy (Fig. 2-2*B*) you can see these synaptic vesicles that have properties matching precisely the requirements for the quantal storage of transmitter preparatory to its emission into the synaptic cleft.

The experiments illustrated in Fig. 2-6 show that not only do you get this *quantal emission* of ACh in the ordinary spontaneous firing, but that nerve impulses also work by liberating quantal packages of transmitter.

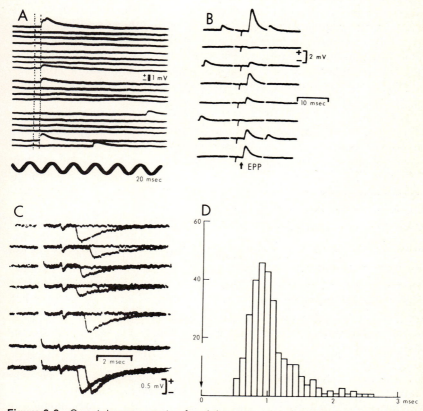

Figure 2-6   Quantal components of endplate potential. *A*. Intracellular recording from frog neuromuscular synapse in calcium-deficient and magnesium-rich medium. Times of nerve stimulus and of EPP onset are indicated by the pair of dotted lines. [*J. del Castillo and B. Katz, J. Physiol.*, **124**:*560 (1954).*] *B*. Intracellular records from a muscle fiber of the rat diaphragm with stimulation of the phrenic nerve (note artifact) also in a calcium-deficient and magnesium-rich medium. [*A. W. Liley, J. Physiol.*, **133**:*571 (1956).*] *C*. Extracellularly recorded EPPs of frog muscle fiber with calcium level adjusted so that only about half the nerve impulses evoked EPPs. *D*. Histogram for latencies of EPPs for the experiment partly illustrated in *C*. [*B. Katz and R. Miledi, Proc. Roy. Soc. B*, **161**:*469 (1965).*]

This quantal composition is not normally revealed in EPPs such as those in Fig. 2-3C because it turns out that some 100 to 200 quanta are liberated by a single nerve impulse at a single endplate, so a "quantal grain" could not be detected. How then can this quantal composition be recognized? If you reduce the amoung of calcium outside the neuromuscular synapse and add a little extra magnesium, you can greatly reduce the effectiveness of the nerve impulse in liberating the transmitter. So it is possible to have endplate potentials of only quantal size. For example, in Fig. 2-6A there are two spontaneous miniature EPPs late in the traces, and slightly later than the nerve impulse (first dotted line) there are three EPPs of about the same size as the spontaneous miniature EPPs, and one in the upper trace that is clearly double. However, in most traces there was no quantal emission. Figure 2-6A is for a frog muscle, while in Fig. 2-6B there is a similar series for a rat muscle. There are five spontaneous miniature EPPs. The EPPs produced by the nerve impulse had a quantal composition of 1, 2, or 3, and there were two examples of failure. The "quantal grain" of the transmitter release stands revealed.

The quantal emission of ACh has been studied in detail and with much ingenuity by Katz and his colleagues and shown to conform exactly with predictions from Poisson's theorem for the independent release of small numbers of quanta. This finding for EPPs as well as the random character of the spontaneous miniature EPPs provide remarkable biological examples of observations that precisely fit predictions from mathematical theory.

In Fig. 2-6C the EPPs are greatly reduced by calcium depletion and are recorded extracellularly as downward deflections. There is a remarkable variance in the EPP latency despite the quite constant latency of the preceding nerve impulse, which is the small diphasic deflection. Evidently the nerve impulse takes very different times to liberate the transmitter, as is more fully illustrated in the histogram of Fig. 2-6D, where there is a surprising range of quantal latencies, 0.5 to 2.5 ms.

The relationship of the nerve impulse to the liberation of the transmitter is shown in Fig. 2-7. In Fig. 2-7A there is the nerve with its branches running along the muscle as in Fig. 2-4, and recording is from two sites on a fine nerve fiber, one (a) near its origin, and the other (b) near its termination. In B and particularly in the very fast records of C you can see that the nerve impulse is recorded at both sites, the distal being later in accordance with a conduction velocity of 0.4 m/s, which is the expected velocity for such a fine unmyelinated fiber.

Figure 2-7D to F further shows that the transmission of the impulse right along the nerve terminal is essential for the effective liberation of the transmitter. Tetrodotoxin (TTX) is employed to block impulse conduction, an action which occurs because of the suppression of the sodium

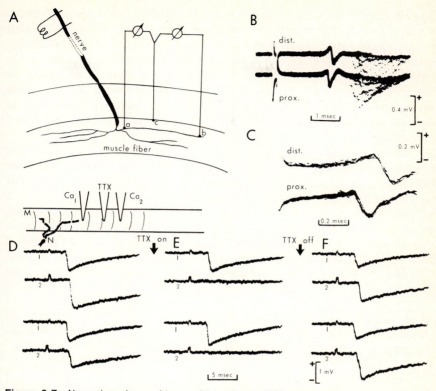

Figure 2-7 Nerve impulse and transmitter release. With stimulating and recording as in *A*, the nerve impulse is recorded in *B* and *C* both at proximal (a) and distal (b) sites on the nerve fiber lying in the groove on the muscle fiber. In *B* are also seen the extracellular EPPs at both distal and proximal recording sites. [*B. Katz and R. Miledi, Proc. Roy. Soc. B, **161**:439 (1965).*] The inset diagram above *D* shows the experimental arrangements for *D* to *F*. N is nerve fiber supplying muscle fiber M, there being three extracellular micropipettes, Ca_1, TTX, and Ca_2 applied at intervals of 93 and 74 μm along a nerve fiber branch lying in a groove on the muscle fiber, but not drawn in as in *A*. The artifacts of the nerve stimulus are seen as a brief upward deflection in all traces of *D* to *F*, and 1 and 2 identify the traces recorded by Ca_1 and Ca_2 micropipettes, respectively. [*B. Katz and R. Miledi, J. Physiol., **199**:729 (1968).*]

conductance mechanism of the impulse as reported in Chap. 1. TTX was applied between two electrodes Ca_1 and Ca_2 of the inset diagram, from which the EPPs of Fig. 2-7*D* to *F* were recorded. When the nerve impulse was blocked, no EPP was recorded at the distal site (*E* 2), but it returned when the TTX block passed off (*F*).

We can conclude first that the impulse normally travels right to the end of the fine nerve fibers and, second, that it is playing a very important role in the liberation of the transmitter (ACh) and the production of the EPP. Actually, other experiments have shown that the nerve impulse is not necessary per se. It is only necessary because of the depolarization which it produces in the presynaptic fiber and which is the essential event triggering the liberation of transmitter. Depolarization by direct electrical means will do as well, as can be demonstrated when the nerve impulse is blocked by TTX. However, propagation of the impulse to the nerve terminal is important because otherwise, as in Fig. 2-7E, the cable properties of the fine nerve terminal are too poor for an effective depolarization to spread for more than a few tens of microns beyond a blocked impulse.

It has already been seen in Fig. 2-6 that synaptic transmission is greatly reduced when calcium is removed from the bathing fluid. For example, in the top trace of Fig. 2-8A the stimulus excites the nerve fiber (see lower diagram), but nothing is recorded from the muscle fiber (m). If a little calcium is injected electrophoretically from the recording micropipette that contains calcium, the nerve impulse is unchanged. But now in the second trace it is liberating quanta of ACh and so produces the small EPP that is recorded extracellularly as a negative wave, just as in Figs. 2-6C and 2-7D to F. A still further calcium injection results in the larger

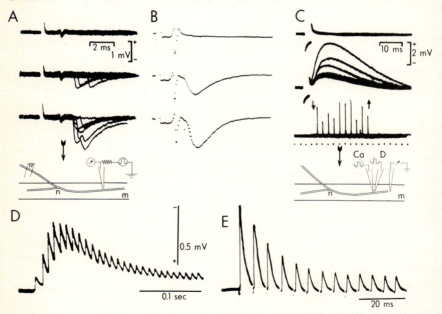

Figure 2-8 Extracellular calcium and neuromuscular transmission. The experimental arrangement for A and B is identified by the arrow below A. The extracellular recording was by a micropipette filled with 0.5 M CaCl₂. [B. Katz and R. Miledi, Proc. Roy. Soc. B, **161**:482 (1965).] The experimental arrangement for C is identified by the arrow below C. [B. Katz and R. Miledi, Proc. Roy. Soc. B, **167**:8 (1967).] D and E are described in the text.

EPP of the third trace of A. In B the averages of 600 successive traces show the graded increase of the EPP from the initial zero, and also that the size of the nerve impulse (the initial diphasic wave indicated by dots) is not affected by the calcium changes.

By contrast calcium is absolutely essential for the release of transmitter from the nerve terminals even in the absence of nerve impulses. In Fig. 2-8C the nerve impulse was blocked by TTX. A depolarizing pulse through electrode D (see inset diagram) was ineffective in the upper frame. In the second frame the electrophoretic injection of Ca^{2+} (see electrode Ca in inset) restored the transmitter release, but with a quantal grain in the size range of the intracellularly recorded EPPs (superimposed traces). The restorative action of the Ca^{2+} injection between the two arrows can be seen in the lowest frame of C at a much slower time scale, where the pulses were applied at the dots at 0.5-s intervals, and the successive EPPs appear as vertical lines.

So far we have concentrated on the action of single impulses at the neuromuscular synapse. However, movements are brought about by repetitive discharge of impulses to muscles, as in Fig. 1-8B. This rapid repetitive activation raises many new problems, of which two are illustrated in Fig. 2-8D and E, where there is recording from the endplate zone of intact muscles. In Fig. 2-8D a curarized frog nerve-muscle preparation was tetanized at 100 per second, and the successive EPPs increased at first and then declined. The reason for the increase appears to be that calcium moved in across the membrane of the nerve terminals (cf. Fig. 2-10) with each impulse in the process of transmitter liberation by that impulse, and that some remained inside and so boosted the transmitter liberation of the next impulse and so on for the several successive impulses at the start. But then the EPPs declined, an effect which is attributed to exhaustion of transmitter, or at least of those synaptic vesicles readily available for ejecting their contents into the synaptic cleft. In Fig. 2-8E with a curarized mammalian preparation there was as usual an immediate decline with no initial phase of calcium potentiation. Evidently transmitter depletion is dominant, but it should be pointed out that the frequency of stimulation (200 per second) is higher than the highest frequencies of discharge of mammalian motoneurons to limb muscles. It has been found that at frequencies above a certain value (about 100 per second) the rate of ACh liberation is constant, the amount per impulse being inversely proportional to frequency.

Hitherto the action of ACh has been investigated by the membrane depolarization produced either by the electrophoretic application of quite large numbers of ACh molecules—about 20 million in Fig. 2-4—or by the quantal emission of some thousands of molecules, as in Figs. 2-5 and 2-6. Recently Katz and Miledi have accomplished a fantastic advance—in fact, to the ultimate level—in their identification of the size and time course of the depolarizations produced by single ACh molecules. This identification is accomplished by spectral frequency analyses of the electrical "noise" that the application of ACh evokes across the postsynaptic membrane (Fig. 2-9A and B). The computer analysis of the noise reveals that it is made up of a random assemblage of extremely minute elements, about $0.3\mu V$, and is of a very brief duration, about 1 ms. It will be recognized that this "noise" is at least 1000 times less than the "biological noise" that was discovered by Fatt and Katz and that turned out to be miniature EPPs. Exquisite testing procedures and rigorous controls establish that these minute potentials are produced by single ACh molecules that momentarily (about 1 ms) attach to receptor sites on the postsynaptic membrane and open ionic gates, presumably by a brief conformational change in the protein structure of the pore (cf. Fig. 1-12). Since the average miniature EPP of frog muscle is about 1500 times larger, it could be concluded that about 1500 ACh molecules participate in generating a miniature EPP and, hence, that there are about 1500 molecules of ACh in a quantum (or synaptic vesicle). However, this would be a minimum number because an appreciable fraction, at least 30 percent of the quantal population, is hydrolyzed by cholinesterase before it can reach a receptor site, as indicated by the ACh-AChE interaction in Fig. 2-10B.

This very interesting and important feature, quantal number, has been studied in a quite different manner by Kuffler and Yoshikami. Bared "craters" of snake neuromuscular junctions were subjected to electrophoretically applied jets (1-ms duration) of ACh. With extremely close apposition the injection produced a depolarization with a remarkable similarity to the miniature EPP, as illustrated in Fig. 2-9C. They utilized a refined biological assay for the estimation of the numbers of ACh molecules actually injected electrophoretically and arrived at a quantal number of 10,000. However, they regard this as an overestimate because the injection site over the "crater" necessarily could not be in such a snug relationship as the nerve terminal. A possible value of 5000 molecules for the snake is not so far removed from the minimum of 1500 molecules derived from Katz and Miledi's results for the frog. On the basis of a quantal number of 5000 and the average size of a miniature EPP (1.5 mV) it can be calculated that a single ACh molecule causes the opening of an ionic channel through which pass 6000 univalent cations in 1 ms. Katz and Miledi calculated a much higher value, 50,000 for the frog, but this is based on the very low estimate of 1000 for the quantal number.

I have given this recent work in some detail because it illustrates so well the advance from neurobiology to molecular neurobiology. It is only 40 years since Dale and his associates made the startling suggestion that neuromuscular transmission was accomplished by the secretion of ACh

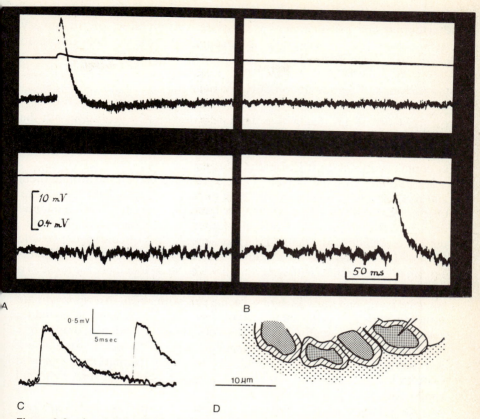

Figure 2-9 *A* and *B*. Intracellular recording from an endplate in frog sartorius at 21°C. In each block, the upper trace was recorded on a low-gain d.c. channel (scale 10 mV); the lower was simultaneously recorded on a high-gain condenser coupled channel (scale 0.4 mV). The top row shows controls (no ACh), the bottom row shows membrane noise during ACh application by diffusion from a micropipette. In the bottom row of records, the increased distance between the low- and high-gain traces is due to upward displacement of the d.c. trace because of ACh-induced depolarization. Two spontaneous min. EPPs are also seen. (*Katz and Miledi, 1972.*) *C* and *D*. Comparison of pipette-evoked ACh potential with min. EPP in a snake muscle fiber. Pulses of 1 ms were passed through an ACh pipette. In *D* the pipette to the right shows the injection site when the boutons were removed, exposing the craters. Two iontophoretically produced responses (left) are superimposed; during one of them a spontaneous min. EPP occurred (right). Rise time (10 to 90 percent) of the response to the pipette-applied ACh is about 1.1 ms, and of the min. EPP about 0.75 ms. The preparation had been lightly treated with collagenase. This treatment removes some, but not all, of the AChE. This accounts for the slightly slower than normal time course of both potentials, although no anticholinesterase was used. (*Kuffler and Yoshikami, 1975b.*)

from the nerve terminals. In addition to the discoveries outlined above this molecular level of investigation has led to a detailed study of the gate-opening times of analogues of ACh and of the effects of temperature, blocking agents, and anticholinesterases. It was not an unexpected finding that curare and prostigmine, for example, had no effect on the unitary ACh action. Those receptors not occupied by curare behaved quite normally to ACh molecules.

Diagrammatic Representation of Neuromuscular Synapses

Figure 2-10A is an imaginative diagram I drew many years ago, but the electron microscope (EM) would still have to be improved by a factor of 10 in order to reveal details like that shown. Meanwhile this diagram is not in conflict with the best EM pictures.

First, there are the synaptic vesicles with the membrane around them and packed tightly inside are the ACh molecules, about 5000 per vesicle. One vesicle is liberating its transmitter into the synaptic cleft—a quantal emission. We do not know how this quantal emission is brought about, only that the influx of calcium ions is essential. And, of course, the vesicle itself is not ejected into the synaptic cleft, only its contents, and then it is assumed to be refilled with acetylcholine and so be available for reuse. To the left is diagrammatically shown a vesicle that has been previously squeezed out and now is being recharged with ACh. An approximate estimate with neuromuscular synapses is that the reserve of synaptic vesicles is only enough for 2000 to 5000 impulses, which is only a few minutes' supply with ordinary muscular activity. Evidently an efficient and fast replenishment is essential. The local new formation of synaptic vesicles or their transport from manufacturing sites in the motoneuronal soma would be much too slow.

Also shown on the postsynaptic membrane of Fig. 2-10A are two types of receptor sites that have different molecular configurations. One type is related to transmembrane channels for ions and these are shown opened up when an ACh molecule is attached. The other type is an acetylcholine esterase site that destroys the attached acetylcholine. A much more detailed and sophisticated diagram of these two types of receptor sites has been published by De Robertis and is shown in Fig. 1-12.

A remarkable new technological advance by De Robertis, Changeux, Barnard, and their associates has led to the identification and even the amino acid sequence of the protein molecules that act specifically as ACh receptors. Furthermore the surface density of these receptor sites has been estimated from a study of the radioactive sites produced when the receptors are combined to the radioactive blocking agent bungarotoxin. There is an amazingly high density of 7000 to 30,000 sites per μm^2. Thus it appears than in 1 μm^2 of the postsynaptic membrane there are enough sites for all of the ACh molecules in a quantum.

Figure 2-10B illustrates other features of the neuromuscular synapse. There is, first, the vesicle with stored ACh, and arrows indicate its release

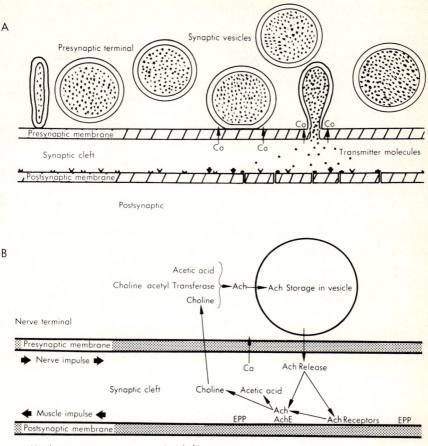

Figure 2-10 Essential elements in neuromusuclar transmission. *A.* Portion of synaptic cleft with synaptic vesicles in close proximity to the presynaptic membrane, one actually discharging transmitter molecules (ACh) into the synaptic cleft. Some molecules are shown combined with receptor sites on the subsynaptic part of postsynaptic membrane with the consequent opening up of pores through that membrane. Arrows denoted Ca show movement of Ca through the presynaptic membrane when it is depolarized. Also shown by different symbols are the molecules of the enzyme acetylcholine esterase attached to the cleft side of the postsynaptic membrane (cf. Fig. 1-12). *B.* Schematic representation of the sequences of events in neuromuscular transmission. Full description in text.

and subsequent fate. Part goes to acetylcholine esterase (AChE) and is very rapidly hydrolyzed into choline and acetic acid, and part goes on to the receptor sites on the postsynaptic membrane, staying there momentarily to open the ionic gates and so produce the endplate potential (EPP). Within 1 to 2 ms it leaves these sites and is rapidly destroyed by the AChE. The effectiveness of this destruction is illustrated in Fig. 2-3*F* and

G where inactivation of the AChE resulted in the large increase of the curarized EPP from *F* to *G*. It is also shown in Fig. 2-5*D*, where the fast-acting anticholinesterase edrophonium caused a large increase in the depolarization produced both by injected ACh and by quantally liberated ACh. Figure 2-10*B* further indicates the operational sequence: ACh on receptor sites; the endplate potential, EPP; the generation of a muscle impulse, the muscle contraction. The diagram, of course, shows only the surface membrane on one side of the muscle fiber.

Also shown in Fig. 2-10*B* is the recycling of choline after it has been produced by hydrolysis of ACh. It diffuses into the nerve terminal and *choline acetyl transferase* combines it with acetic acid to reform ACh in the cytoplasm. Pumping into the synaptic vesicles replenishes their ACh stores and so completes the cycle.

The key factor in the emission of ACh by the vesicles is the entry of calcium into the presynaptic terminal (Fig. 2-10*A*). Because the quantal release of ACh is approximately proportional to the fourth power of the external Ca^{2+} concentration it has been postulated that 4 Ca^{2+} ions are necessary for one vesicle to burst. In order to have this concentration of Ca^{2+} ions in proximity to one vesicle it is necessary to have an immense excess of entering calcium—actually about 10,000 times as much. Even with the large excess there is often a little delay in the assemblage of the necessary 4 Ca^{2+} ions, which presumably accounts for the variability in the timing of quantal emission in Figs. 2-6*C* and *D* and 2-8*A*.

Figure 2-11 gives a more detailed diagram of the events occurring in neuromuscular transmission with special reference to the ionic mechanisms. In Fig. 2-11*A* there is shown a nerve terminal with the vesicles in position, the synaptic cleft and the postsynaptic membrane. In Fig. 2-11*B* the part framed by the dotted line is enlarged and the various kinds of ionic channels with their gates are shown, much as in Fig. 1-15 for nerve impulse propagation. Na_D and K_D depict the sodium and potassium channels for the impulse, the subscript D indicating that depolarization opens their gates. Na_D and K_D are shown along the whole length of the nerve terminal, because the impulse propagation in these terminal fibers has been shown in Fig. 2-7*B* and *C*. In addition, there are also special Ca_D channels with gates in the nerve terminal, also with the D subscript. It takes about 30 mV depolarization to begin the opening of a Na_D gate (Fig. 1-14), and it is about the same for a Ca_D gate. Despite this similarity they are quite distinct, as is shown, for example, by the action of TTX in blocking Na_D and leaving Ca_D unaltered. When the Ca_D gate is opened, Ca^{2+} ions rapidly diffuse in down their electrochemical gradient, which is very large (almost 200 mV), and so are able to cause emission from the vesicles.

Figure 2-11*B* further illustrates the ionic mechanism of the postsynaptic membrane. The transmitter acts on the receptor sites illustrated in

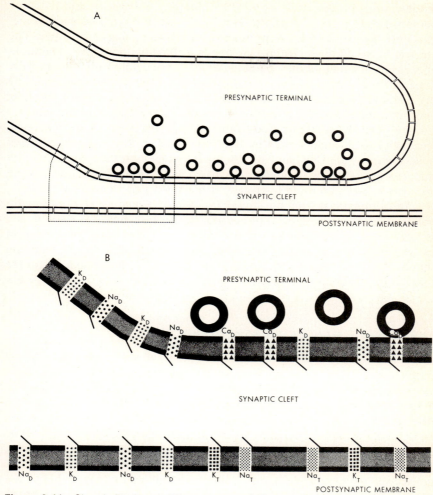

Figure 2-11 Chemically transmitting synapse. *A.* Presynaptic terminal separated by the synaptic cleft from postsynaptic membrane, and containing many spherical synaptic vesicles, some close to the membrane fronting the synaptic cleft. Note the various channels through the membrane. *B.* Segment outlined by the broken line in *A* is shown enlarged to give fine detail. Note that all channels have a gate control, and that symbols in the channels indicate five different kinds of chemical constitution for the carrier molecules: Na_D, K_D, Ca_D, Na_T, K_T. The subscripts D and T indicate opening by depolarization, and by the transmitter substance, respectively.

Fig. 2-10*A*. In Fig. 2-11*B* there are special sites for potassium and sodium ions, labeled K_T and Na_T. The subscript T signifies their opening by transmitter. Depolarization is without effect on their opening. The existence of these two kinds of ionic gates and associated channels as distinct entities has been supported by experiments by the Takeuchi's on the modifications produced in the EPP by changes both in the external ionic composition and in the potential across the postsynaptic membrane. Probably these channels are preferential and not exclusive as drawn. The electric currents through the Na_T and K_T channels normally balance at about -15-mV membrane potential, which is the equilibrium potential for the EPP, Fig. 2-3B. This value is a compromise between a value of $+50$ mV for the Na_T channel and -99 mV for the K_T channel for the frog neuromuscular synapse. It will be noted that in Fig. 2-11B the Na_T and K_T channels are sharply restricted to the postsynaptic membrane in accordance with experiments such as that illustrated in Fig. 2-4. Beyond that zone there are the Na_D and K_D channels resembling those in nerve and that likewise are operatively concerned with the propagation of the impulse along the muscle fiber after it has been generated by the EPP.

In summary it can be stated that Figs. 2-10 and 2-11 pictorially display the essential features of neuromuscular transmission in so far as it is understood at the present time. Furthermore it will be shown that in essential operational features these diagrams also help in understanding the mechanisms of synaptic transmission in the brain, though of course other transmitters are there concerned.

TRANSMISSION ACROSS THE GIANT SYNAPSE IN THE STELLATE GANGLION OF THE SQUID

In Chap. 1, investigations of the squid giant axon were of fundamental importance. Here we are going to describe experiments on the giant synapse in the stellate ganglion from which the giant fiber arises (Fig. 1-10A). In the diagram of Fig. 2-12H there is shown the large presynaptic fiber (Pre) making a giant-sized synaptic contact with the postsynaptic fiber (Post), which is the giant fiber utilized in the experiments described in the first chapter. The advantage of this synapse is that it is very large. The presynaptic and postsynaptic fibers are several hundred microns across and the region of synaptic contact is a millimeter long, although the actual synaptic contacts are patchy. This synapse gives unique opportunities for investigation. For example, electrodes can be inserted into the presynaptic fiber for direct recording of its membrane potential and its action potential, or for passing currents to alter the membrane potential, a facility that is not possible with the neuromuscular synapse because the presynaptic nerve terminal is far too small.

The giant synapse qualifies on all tests as a chemical synapse. There is a synaptic delay of about 1 ms, a value much like the neuromuscular synapse. There are typical synaptic vesicles, a synaptic cleft and spontaneous quantal emission to give miniature synaptic potentials. The transmitter is not acetylcholine. It is probably glutamate or a near chemical relative.

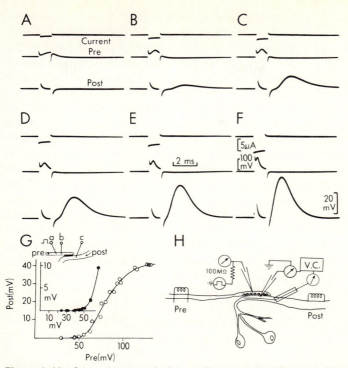

Figure 2-12 Synaptic transmission, stellate ganglion. Presynaptic depolarization and transmitter release with impulses eliminated by TTX. *H* is a drawing of the whole synaptic structure of the stellate ganglion of the squid (cf. Fig. 1-10), with experimental arrangements. Pre: presynaptic terminal. Post: postsynaptic giant axon. In the upper diagram of *G* are the special arrangements for this experiment. Length of synaptic contact, 0.8 mm. a: current-passing electrode; b: prerecording electrode; c: postrecording electrode. *A-F.* Sample recordings in six frames: upper trace, applied current pulse; middle and lower, presynaptic and postsynaptic potentials recorded through electrodes b and c, respectively. *G.* Input-output relation obtained with 1-ms current pulses. Abscissa, peak of presynaptic depolarization; ordinate, size of postsynaptic response. Inset, initial part of curve in greater detail. Temperature in these experiments was about 10°C; concentration of tetrodotoxin 2×10^{-7} g/ml. [*B. Katz and R. Miledi, Nature, 212:1242 (1966).*]

Figure 2-12 illustrates a remarkable experiment by Katz and Miledi which shows the way in which the large dimensions of this giant synapse can be utilized to disclose special features of chemical synaptic transmission. Impulse transmission was blocked by TTX and presynaptic depolarization was effected by intracellular application of a brief current pulse (see *a* in inset of *G*), as shown in the upper traces of the series of frames *A* through *F*. Below are shown the presynaptic (Pre) and postsynaptic (Post) membrane potentials. In *A* the presynaptic depolarization had no postsynaptic effect, there being only brief artifacts at "on" and "off." In *B* there was a slight depolarizing action and in C to F it did more and more. The plotted points in G show that the more you depolarize the terminal (plotted as abscissas) the more transmitter is liberated, as indicated by the postsynaptic depolarization (ordinates). However, there had to be almost 40 mV presynaptic depolarization before any transmitter was liberated— note the more sensitive plotting in the inset of G.

Figure 2-13 illustrates essentially the same results under conditions where presynaptic currents were employed to change the size of the presynaptic impulse in a preparation not poisoned by TTX. In the frame labeled 0, no current was passed and the large presynaptic action potential (upper trace) evoked a later postsynaptic potential like an endplate potential. It is called a synaptic potential or, in accordance with usual terminology, an excitatory postsynaptic potential, EPSP. When the presynaptic impulse was increased by making the membrane potential larger, the output of transmitter was increased, as indicated by the EPSPs in the frames labeled +3 to +8. If, on the other hand, the presynaptic impulse was decreased by reducing the membrane potential (frames −3 to −9), the EPSPs reveal that the liberation of transmitter was reduced even to zero.

It is a remarkable finding in Figs. 2-12 and 2-13 that a threshold depolarization of about 40 mV is necessary for transmitter liberation from the presynaptic terminal. This can be regarded as the threshold for opening the calcium gates on the presynaptic terminal so that Ca^{2+} can enter the presynaptic terminal (cf. the Ca_D gates in Fig. 2-11). Just as with the neuromuscular synapses, there is direct experimental evidence that the influx of Ca^{2+} ions is essential for the quantal liberation of the transmitter, as has been diagrammed in Figs. 2-10A and 2-11B. When the Ca^{2+} of the bathing fluid was greatly reduced, synaptic transmission was blocked just as with the neuromuscular synapse (Fig. 2-8A, B, C). It is restored by injection of Ca^{2+} ions close to the external surface of the synapse even at a rate as low as 10^{-14} to 10^{-15} mole of Ca^{2+} ions in 1 s. The role of Ca^{2+} ions in causing the emission of transmitter has recently been elegantly displayed by Miledi who has injected Ca^{2+} ions electrophoretically into the presynaptic terminal in a preparation pretreated by TTX. The Ca^{2+} injection results in an enormous output of transmitter, which is in the form of a quantal release.

We can now summarize the findings on the giant synapse by returning to Fig. 2-11. The Ca^{2+} gates only start to open when there is about 40 mV depolarization, but with 80 or 100 mV they must be much more widely open. Under such conditions there is an influx of more calcium and therefore more vesicles discharge. The curve of Fig. 2-12G shows that transmitter liberation increases further with membrane potential changes up to 150 mV, i.e., with a large reversal of membrane potential. One other feature of the squid giant synapse is that the action of

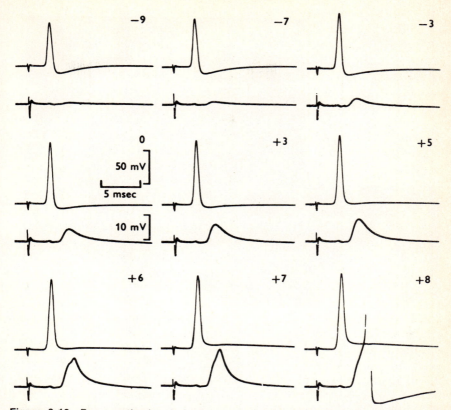

Figure 2-13 Presynaptic depolarization and transmitter release. The experimental arrangements are shown in Fig. 2-12*H*. Prolonged currents of the intensities indicated for each frame in relative units were passed through the electrode inserted into the presynaptic element. This electrode was also used for recording the presynaptic action potentials (upper traces of each frame) evoked by a presynaptic stimulus (note stimulus artifact). The lower traces are the simultaneously recorded postsynaptic responses. [*R. Miledi and C. R. Slater, J. Physiol., **184**:473 (1966).*]

the transmitter on the postsynaptic membrane is almost exclusively to open the Na_T channels. Thus Gage and Moore found that the equilibrium potential for the EPSP was almost as positive as for Na^+ ions. If Fig. 2-11*B* were to represent a squid giant synapse, it would be necessary to delete most of the K_T channels.

TRANSMISSION ACROSS SYNAPSES ON GANGLION CELLS IN THE FROG HEART

This investigation of Kuffler and his colleagues is of great importance because for the first time it was possible to carry out precise investigations on synapses that could be visualized in the living state. In Fig. 2-14

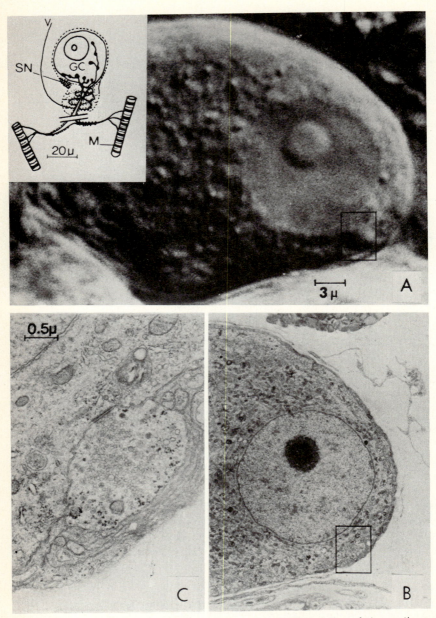

Figure 2-14 Synapses on ganglion cell in frog auricle. Correlation of observations on living cells with electron microscopy. Inset diagram shows ganglion cell, GC, with axon distributed to cardiac muscle fibers M, and with presynaptic vagal fiber, V, approaching the cell in a spiral. *A.* Living nerve cell body and the outline of a synaptic bouton (box) seen with Nomarski optics. *B.* Same neuron prepared for electron microscopy and serially sectioned in the appropriate plane for comparison with corresponding

the inset diagram shows a single ganglion cell, GC, with its nucleus and nucleolus. The vagal fiber (V) comes in, spirals around the cell's axon and makes synapses, shown as little dark knobs, on the cell body. There are no dendrites. The cell's axon goes out to cardiac muscle fibers, M, and inhibits them. Both the vagal synapses on the cell and the cell's axon on cardiac muscle have acetylcholine (ACh) as the transmitter, the latter being the chemical transmitter action originally discovered by Loewi in the 1920s.

In Fig. 2-14A there is a high magnification of such a ganglion cell as it is revealed in optical section by the high resolution given in Nomarski interference microscopy. Most of the same ganglion cell is shown at the same magnification in B, the nucleus and nucleolus serving as orientation features. Finally in C there is a high magnification of the electron micrograph of B. In C there is a good display of a synaptic knob filled with vesicles and with a synaptic cleft partly specialized as a darker staining active site (cf. Fig. 1-4B). This synapse can be identified as the ill-defined structure framed by the rectangle in A, which is drawn identically with that in B. With much experience and checking by electron micrographs as in B and C, or by stained preparations, it has been possible to identify synapses in the living state with assurance.

Figure 2-15 illustrates an elegant experiment that is possible with this isolated ganglion cell. It is a most impressive demonstration of the way in which electrophoretically applied ACh can mimic excitation by a synapse in which ACh is the transmitter. In the first column of Fig. 2-15 are the responses produced by three different electrophoretic applications of ACh in close proximity to a visualized synapse, as in Fig. 2-4. The upper traces give the intracellular recording of the cell response, the lower the brief currents (one marked by arrow) that are electrophoretically applying the ACh to the synapse. In C the application produced only a synaptic depolarization, much as in Fig. 2-4C, but in A and B the larger applications of ACh resulted in larger synaptic potentials that generated an impulse discharge. In the second column are the responses evoked by an impulse in the vagal fiber (V in the inset of Fig. 2-14). In D the response is under resting conditions, with the excitatory postsynaptic potential (EPSP) so large that it was fused with the immediately generated impulse discharge. There was a later prolonged depolarization that can be attributed to the continued action of the transmitter, just as with the hump in the action potential of Fig. 2-3B at the endplate region. It is closely mimicked by the largest ACh injection (A). With continuation of the nerve stimulation there was depletion of transmitter (cf. Fig 2-8D and E),

landmarks seen in A at the same magnification. C. Higher EM magnification of the synaptic region reveals structures typical for chemical synapses, synaptic vesicles, and a patch of densely staining membranes on either side of the synaptic cleft. (*From U. J. McMahan and S. W. Kuffler, 1971.*)

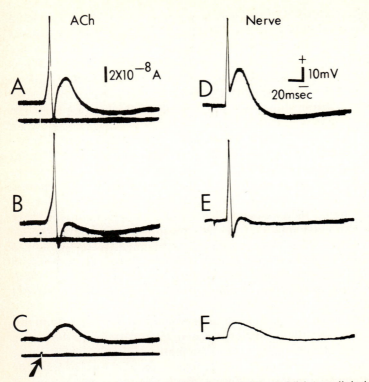

Figure 2-15 Responses of frog ganglion cell (Fig. 2-14) intracellularly recorded and evoked by electrophoretic application of ACh and by nerve stimulation. *A, B*, and *C* are evoked by progressively smaller current pulses (1 ms duration) through the extracellular micropipette filled with a strong solution of ACh. *D, E*, and *F* are synaptically evoked by a single preganglionic nerve impulse (note time of stimulus artifacts). *D* is the initial response of a repetitive train of stimuli, *E* and *F* are later when the emission of ACh is progressively reduced. (*From Dennis, Harris, and Kuffler, 1971.*)

but in *E* there was still sufficient to produce an EPSP that generated an impulse discharge, though there was only a small later depolarization. The nerve impulse is here mimicking the response produced by the ACh injection in *B*. After further transmitter depletion a nerve impulse produced an EPSP too small to initiate an impulse, *F*, closely resembling *C*. The close correspondence between the two series gives a beautiful display of the way in which the electrophoretic application of acetylcholine matches the neural application, there being approximately a 10-fold discrepancy in the amounts required.

Figure 2-16 gives an illustration of the potentialities of this remarkable preparation. All traces are intracellular recordings from the same ganglion cell. The lowest trace shows, at the normal membrane potential, the responses evoked both by an electrophoretic application of ACh and by a nerve stimulation that was reduced as in Fig. 2-15F so that it gave only a synaptic potential. In the remainder of the series the membrane potential was changed by the outward passage of a steady current, at four levels of intensity. The ordinate scale represents the membrane potential. It can be seen that the potentials produced by the acetylcholine application, both electrophoretic and neural, were firstly reduced, then abolished, then reversed. There was a remarkable parallel at all levels of membrane potential, and for both the reversal potential was shown to be at about −2 mV when the whole series was plotted.

CONCLUDING STATEMENTS

We have finished the story of the investigations on peripheral synapses. In the principal example a nerve impulse propagates to the nerve terminals of a synapse and there acts with extraordinary efficiency and speed to inject acetylcholine into the exceedingly narrow cleft between the nerve fiber and the muscle fiber. The electrical activity of the nerve impulse has been transformed into a chemical injection. Then in turn the chemical transmitter momentarily opens ionic gates on the postsynaptic

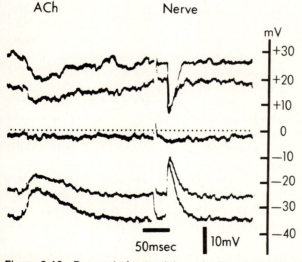

Figure 2-16 Reversal of potentials evoked by electrophoretic application of ACh, and by synaptic transmission. Same preparation as in Fig. 2-15, but membrane potential of the ganglion cell was changed by progressively increasing outwardly directed currents. It was possible to reverse the membrane potential and the evoked responses were also reversed (uppermost traces) to become virtual mirror images of the responses at the resting potential (lowest trace). (*From Dennis, Harris, and Kuffler, 1971.*)

membrane, and so reconstitutes an electrical process—an endplate potential leading on to a muscle impulse—on the far side of the synapse. It may be asked: What is the point of this double transformation? Could not the electric energy of the nerve impulse be utilized to excite the muscle fiber directly? The answer is easy and obvious. There is large electrical mismatch between the very fine nerve fiber and the large muscle fiber, which means that the currents responsible for the propagation of the nerve impulse (cf. Fig. 1-16) would be far too small to excite the muscle fiber no matter how efficiently the nerve-muscle junction would be arranged. The chemical transmitting mechanism overcomes this extreme disability by introducing an amplification of an order larger than 100-fold. In fact there is a safety factor of about 5 in transmission from nerve impulses to muscle fibers. This is a very important safeguard for our muscular performance even under extreme conditions, when, for example, the supply of transmitter may be depleted. Muscle remains a reliable servant in carrying out the commands of the nervous system, as is illustrated in Fig. 2-1.

The vital significance of this reliability is brought home to one when failure threatens. In a disease called *myasthenia gravis* the amounts of acetylcholine produced are reduced and the replenishment is not fast enough. So with a little exertion the patient becomes greatly weakened or even paralyzed. For this reason it is a very serious and even fatal disease. The treatment is not yet satisfactory, but, by giving an anticholinesterase such as prostigmine, the optimum conditions are provided for the patients to make the most of the acetylcholine that they can produce. But of course the real challenge in combating this disease is to discover the factors which result in the deficiency of ACh production.

The weakening of neuromuscular transmission by curare has already been mentioned as a valuable help in surgery. Recovery after the operation is speeded by an injection of anticholinesterase that prevents the transmitter (ACh) from being destroyed by AChE. Consequently more is available for overcoming the continuing curare blockade.

It is of interest that neuromuscular synapses are very sensitive to one of the most poisonous substances known, botulinum toxin. Botulinum toxin is extremely powerful in preventing the nerve endings from liberating acetylcholine and so it kills by muscular paralysis—breathing becomes impossible.

These illustrations serve to show that, even though chemical synaptic transmission is a beautifully designed biological mechanism, it has inherent disabilities and dangers. In the next chapter there will be an account of chemical synapses in the brain, where we shall see that they are essential for the operation of complex nervous systems. The alternative synaptic mechanism, by electrical transmission, apparently is used only at special sites in the brains of lower animals (where accurate timing is essential) and not to any significant extent in the mammalian brain.

REFERENCES

Dale, H. H. (1938): "Acetylcholine as a Chemical Transmitter Substance of the Effects of Nerve Impulses," The William Henry Welch Lectures, 1937, *J. Mt. Sinai Hosp.*, **4**:401–429.

Dennis, M. J., A. J. Harris, and S. W. Kuffler (1971): "Synaptic Transmission and Its Duplication by Focally Applied Acetylcholine in Parasympathetic Neurons in the Heart of the Frog," *Proc. Roy. Soc. B*, **177**:509–539.

De Robertis, E. (1975): *Synaptic Receptors. Isolation and Molecular Biology*, Marcel Dekker, New York.

Eccles, J. C. (1964): *The Physiology of Synapses*, Springer, Berlin, Göttingen, and Heidelberg.

Eccles, J. C. (1966): "The Ionic Mechanisms of Excitatory and Inhibitory Synaptic Action," *Ann. N.Y. Acad. Sci.*, **137**:473–495.

Gage, P. W., and J. W. Moore (1969): "Synaptic Current at the Squid Giant Synapse," *Science*, **160**:510–512.

Hubbard, J. I. (1970): "Mechanism of Transmitter Release," *Progr. Biophys. Mol. Biol.*, **21**:33–124.

Hubbard, J. I. (ed.) (1974): *The Peripheral Nervous System*, Plenum, New York.

Katz, B. (1962): "The Transmission of Impulses from Nerve to Muscle, and the Subcellular Unit of Synaptic Action," *Proc. Roy. Soc. B*, **155**:455–479.

Katz, B. (1966): *Nerve, Muscle, and Synapse*, McGraw-Hill, New York.

Katz, B. (1969): *The Release of Neural Transmitter Substances*, Liverpool University Press, Liverpool.

Katz, B., and R. Miledi (1972): "The Statistical Nature of the Acetylcholine Potential and Its Molecular Components," *J. Physiol.*, **224**:665–699.

Katz, B., and R. Miledi (1973): "The Binding of Acetylcholine to Receptors and Its Removal from the Synaptic Cleft," *J. Physiol.*, **231**:549–574.

Kuffler, S. W., and D. Yoshikami (1975a): "The Distribution of Acetylcholine Sensitivity at the Postsynaptic Membrane of Vertebral Skeletal Twitch Muscles: Iontophoretic Mapping in the Micron Range," *J. Physiol.*, **244**:703–730.

Kuffler, S. W., and D. Yoshikami (1975b): "The Number of Transmitter Molecules in a Quantum: An Estimate from Iontophoretic Application of Acetylcholine at the Neuromuscular Synapse," *J. Physiol.*, **251**:465–482.

McMahan, U. J., and S. W. Kuffler (1971): "Visual Identification of Synaptic Boutons on Living Ganglion Cells and of Varicosities in Postganglionic Axons in the Heart of the Frog," *Proc. Roy. Soc. B*, **177**:485–508.

McMahan, U. J., N. C. Spitzer, and K. Pepper (1972): "Visual Identification of Nerve Terminals in Living Isolated Skeletal Muscle," *Proc. Roy. Soc. B*, **181**:421–430.

Martin, A. R. (1966): "Quantal Nature of Synaptic Transmission," *Physiol. Rev.*, **46**:51–66.

Miledi, D. (1973): "Transmitter Release Induced by Injection of Calcium Ions into Nerve Terminals," *Proc. Roy. Soc. B*, **183**:421–425.

Miledi, D., and C. R. Slater (1966): "The Action of Calcium on Neuronal Synapses in the Squid," *J. Physiol.*, **184**:473–498.

Peper, K., and U. J. McMahan (1972): "Distribution of Acetylcholine Receptors in the Vicinity of Nerve Terminals on Skeletal Muscle of the Frog," *Proc. Roy. Soc. B*, **181**:431–440.

Synaptic Transmission and Pathways in the Brain

SYNAPTIC PATHWAYS AND SYNAPTIC STRUCTURE

Figure 2-1 introduces the problems of this chapter. In the first chapter there was an account of conduction of the nerve impulse, in the second transmission across the neuromuscular junction and of the concept of the motor unit. Motor units are the executive units whereby the brain gains expression in movement. As I explained in Chap. 2, all actions are effected by the firing of impulses by motoneurons. When there is this firing in response to instructions from the brain, the motor unit acts as a perfect servant of the brain.

The first question in this chapter is: What makes the motoneuron fire? Let us start with two simple reflex pathways (Fig. 1-6) that were drawn long ago by Ramón y Cajal and that we briefly considered in Chap. 1. The simplest reflex arc shown in Fig. 1-6A has been of great importance in investigations of the central nervous system. In the muscle is a stretch receptor (cf. Fig. 1-8A) located on a special type of muscle fiber (cf. Fig. 4-7) and called the *annulospiral ending* because of its shape, labeled AS, in the insets of Fig. 3-1A. In a large muscle there are of course hundreds of muscle spindles with annulospiral endings, each with a large afferent fiber of a special type—group Ia. When you stretch the muscle by a brief tap to the tendon at the knee joint, impulses pass up the Ia afferent fibers into the spinal cord and so directly to motoneurons (Fig. 3-1A) that are excited to fire impulses out to the muscle which is caused to contract. That is a knee jerk. If, alternatively, you stretch the muscle slowly and then keep it stretched, the annulospiral endings will continue discharging impulses as illustrated in Fig. 1-8A and the muscle will give a slow postural or tonic contraction.

In Fig. 1-6B is a more complicated reflex pathway. To the right is a cutaneous receptor whose responses have been illustrated in Chap. 1 (Fig. 1-7A), where it was stimulated by touch or pressure on the skin. The afferent fiber passes into the spinal cord just as in A, but it branches a great deal and the pathway to motoneurons is always via interneurons, only one of which is shown. Actually there are enormous numbers of interneurons, with many arranged in parallel, but they also are serially arranged so that the reflex is a very wide spreading and prolonged response of the muscles. A simple example of such a reflex occurs if you touch something unexpectedly hot. You will find that you withdraw your hand before you feel the pain. It is the same if you step on some sharp

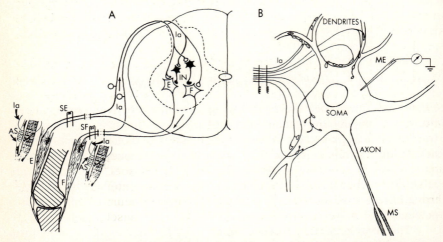

Figure 3-1 Simple reflex pathways and responses. *A* is a diagrammatic representation of the pathways from and to the extensor (E) and flexor (F) muscles of the knee joint. The small insets show the details of the origin of the Ia afferent fibers from the annulospiral endings (AS) of muscle spindles. *B* is a detail showing the many Ia synapses on a motoneuron. Full description in text.

object. You will withdraw your leg by contracting all your flexor muscles acting at all the different joints, as illustrated by the three sets of muscles in Fig. 1-6B. This rapid unconscious withdrawal is effected by pathways in the spinal cord. At the same time impulses pass up the spinal cord to the higher levels of your brain (cf. Fig. 3-13) and tell you what is happening, but of course this information is experienced after the reflex withdrawal has occurred.

Sherrington's classic book *The Integrative Action of the Nervous System* dealt with systems like this and some that were more complicated. In fact the whole basis for our understanding of the neuronal machinery of the brain derives from his classical contributions and discoveries, for which he was awarded the Nobel prize in 1932. I will briefly describe two of his important concepts. First is the *principle of divergence*, whereby one afferent fiber coming into the spinal cord and carrying its own specific message diverges to many lines activating many nerve cells, as illustrated in Fig. 1-6A and B. Second, there is the complementary *principle of convergence*, whereby not only is there this wide dispersion of information but also onto each nerve cell in the brain there is convergence of many lines of impulse traffic. As a simple example, in the diagram of Fig. 3-1A, it should be shown that the Ia fibers from many other stretch receptors in the muscle converge onto each of the motoneurons innervating that muscle (Fig. 3-1B). It is the same with all other reflex pathways. All are made up of these diverging and converging lines, which are not only on the final path from motoneuron to muscle, but at the various interneurons on the way. Convergence onto a neuron is diagrammatically shown in Fig. 1-3A for a standard kind of neuron with soma and the stumps of the dendrites and axon.

In Fig. 3-1A the afferent fiber (Ia) from the annulospiral ending (AS) of the knee extensor muscle (E) enters a dorsal root of the spinal cord and acts directly on a motoneuron (E) of that muscle. *It should be recognized that there are many hundreds of lines in parallel to the one drawn, giving immense scope for divergence and convergence.*

The antagonist muscle is the flexor (F) that bends the leg back at the knee. In this muscle there are the same annulospiral receptor organs (AS) and the motor endplates made by the motor nerve fiber. Impulses from the stretch receptors (AS) of the flexor muscle also enter the spinal cord through the dorsal root and directly excite the motoneuron (F), innervating the flexor muscle. So the extensor and flexor muscles have central pathways complementary to each other.

In addition there is a reciprocal arrangement in Fig. 3-1A. The afferent fiber from the extensor muscle (E) branches in the spinal cord so that not only does it excite its own motoneuron, but it also sends a branch which excites an interneuron (IN). This neuron is shown in black and it sends its axon to the antagonist motoneuron (F) and forms inhibitory synapses on it. (Throughout this book I will use in diagrams the symbols black for inhibition and white for excitation.) In the same way there is the reciprocal arrangement for the afferent fibers from the flexor muscles acting on inhibitory neurons to extensor motoneurons.

This very simple reciprocal arrangement can be given functional meaning. When you are standing with slightly bent knees your weight is stretching the knee extensor muscle (E) and the AS stretch receptors are firing into the spinal cord, exciting the knee extensor motoneurons to fire impulses so that the extensor muscle contracts and holds your weight. If this muscle contraction is inadequate, the knee gives a little, so stretching the extensor muscle more, with more firing from its AS receptors giving an increased reflex discharge to the muscle, which in this way is nicely adjusted to give a steady posture. At the same time the reciprocal inhibitory pathway prevents the antagonist motoneurons (F) from firing to give contraction of the antagonist flexor muscles (F). Such a contraction would oppose the extensors that are engaged in the essential task of weight supporting. This description of the mode of action of the pathways in Fig. 3-1A illustrates a simple reflex performance.

SYNAPTIC EXCITATORY ACTION

Figure 3-1B is a drawing of a motoneuron in the cat's spinal cord with its axon gaining a myelin sheath (MS) as seen in Fig. 1-4A. The dendrites are truncated and several synaptic knobs are shown. In addition, on the right is shown a microelectrode (ME) inserted into the soma, which we first did in 1951 following the procedure of Fatt and Katz the year before in their classic investigation on the neuromuscular synapse (Fig. 2-3A to C). A motoneuron such as that of Fig. 3-1B is about 70 μm across. The fine glass tube used as the microelectrode was only half a micron (0.0005 mm) across at its tip, and it was filled with conducting salt solution (3 M KCl). It is drawn magnified about five times relative to the neuron. It was a nice discovery that, if you penetrate the cell membrane with such fine glass tubes of a very gradual taper and carefully protect them from mechanical vibrations, they will self-seal in the membrane and give a steady and reliable method of leading from the interior of the cell against the surround on which is placed the indifferent or ground electrode. In this way all potential changes across the surface membrane of the neuron are recorded on the oscilloscope after suitable amplification. Thus you have a direct recording of synaptic action on the surface membrane, just as was done in the simpler situations of the neuromuscular junction, the squid synapse, and the frog ganglion cell in Chap. 2.

In Fig. 3-1B a number of Ia afferent fibers from annulospiral endings are drawn making monosynaptic connections, as we say, because there is only one synapse on the way from the muscle receptors to the moto-neuron innervating the muscle. A stimulating electrode is shown to the left on the seven Ia fibers, but in our experiments (cf. Fig. 3-2) it was on the nerve to the muscle innervated by the motoneuron in which there would be 100 or so such fibers. By gradually increasing the strength of this nerve stimulation you cause more and more nerve fibers to fire single impulses up to the spinal cord and so to the synapses of this motoneuron.

In Fig. 3-2 the upper traces of the frames *A* to *I* show the action potentials of these Ia afferent fibers with the increasing size as the stimulus was increased to excite more of them. Correspondingly, in the lower traces of each frame there is a progressive increase in the more prolonged potentials that look like the endplate potentials produced by neuromuscular synapses (Fig. 2-3*C*, *F*, and *G*) when transmission is depressed by curare or calcium deficiency. These potentials in the

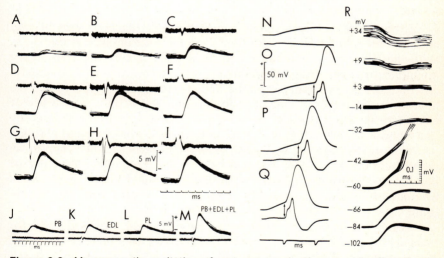

Figure 3-2 Monosynaptic excitation of motoneurons by the group Ia afferent path-way. In *A* to *I* the upper traces give the size of the afferent volley as it enters the spinal cord, and the lower the simultaneously recorded EPSPs. All records are formed by the superposition of about 25 faint traces. In *J* to *L* the EPSPs are recorded in another motoneuron (peroneus longus) in response to maximum group I volleys in the nerves to three muscles, peroneus brevis, extensor digitorum longus, and peroneus longus, and in *M* to all three combined. [*J. C. Eccles, R. M. Eccles, and A. Lundberg, J. Physiol.,* **136**:527 (1957).] *N* to *Q* illustrate graded responses in another motoneuron with the generation of an impulse discharge to *O* to *Q*. The differentiated records in the lower traces show its double composition, the impulse being generated first in the axonal region of Fig. 3-1*B*. In *R* are a series of EPSPs (superimposed faint traces) recorded when the membrane potential of the motoneuron (initially 66 mV) was set at the indicated levels by the passage of a steady current through the intracellular microelec-trode. [*J. C. Coombs, J. C. Eccles, and P. Fatt, J. Physiol.,* **130**:174 (1955).]

depolarizing direction are produced by excitatory synapses and are called *excitatory postsynaptic potentials (EPSP)*. The increase in size from *A* to *F* is due to convergence onto this motoneuron of progressively more Ia impulses with their excitatory synapses. Within limits there is a linear summation of the EPSPs produced by each synapse. For example, *J, K,* and *L* show EPSPs by three independent sets of excitatory synapses on a motoneuron, and in *M* superposition results in an EPSP which is almost exactly the sum of these three individually. This so-called *spatial summation* is what you would expect theoretically. When there are many synapses converging on a neuron, each of them exerts its synaptic action to take charge off the membrane and so to excite the neuron.

In Fig. 3-2*A* to *M* the EPSPs were not adequate to excite the neuron to fire impulses. However in another experiment (Fig. 3-2*N* to *Q*) this did occur. The millisecond scale shows that the sweep speed was about five times faster and the amplification was about one-seventh. When allowance is made for these different conditions of recording, Fig. 3-2*N* is seen to be an EPSP rather like the larger EPSPs of 3-2*D* to *I*. With a slight strengthening of the nerve stimulus in *O* the EPSP reached a critical level and fired an impulse, just as the EPP fired a muscle impulse in Fig. 2-3*B*. With the still larger EPSPs in *P* and *Q* the firing occurred earlier, at the double arrows. The firing of an impulse can be regarded as a successful outcome of the excitatory synaptic action. If the EPSPs fail to fire the neuron, they have been made for no purpose. But if the convergence of excitatory input is adequate to fire a neuron, the impulse discharged by that neuron travels along all the axon branches. For example, if it is a motoneuron, the impulse will traverse all the branches to the synapses on the muscle fibers (cf. Fig. 2-1), which is an example of the principle of divergence. With neurons other than motoneurons the divergence would be onto the neurons next in series in all the complex pathways of the brain.

Though summation of unitary EPSPs to reach a critical level for firing an impulse is the normal mode of operation, this same result can be achieved by any depolarizing process. For example, if a steady current is applied to the neuron, depolarizing it to some level short of the firing level, a superimposed EPSP has a correspondingly easier task in firing an impulse. In Fig. 3-2*O* to *Q* the membrane potential was −70 mV and the critical level for firing an impulse was −52 mV, which could be by the EPSP or by any combination of background depolarization and EPSP.

In Fig. 1-4*A* (giant boutons) and *B* to the left there are examples of large excitatory synapses such as the ones presumed to be activated by the stretch receptors of a muscle in Figs. 3-1 and 4-7. In Fig. 1-4*B* the arrow points to the narrow *synaptic cleft* between the synaptic knob and the surface of the neuron on which it is ending. There are the numerous spherical synaptic vesicles and also the mitochondrion—much as in the larger neuromuscular synapse (Fig. 2-2B). At the neuromuscular synapse the single synapse has to fire a muscle impulse or it has failed operationally. On the other hand, there are hundreds and even thousands of synapses for the convergent pathways onto a single neuron. In fact, one type of neuron, the Purkinje cell (PC in Fig. 4-11), has about 80,000 of these excitatory synaptic endings, but they are small. In Figs. 1-4B and 1-5 the vesicles are clustered along most of the synaptic surface and there is the characteristic density of the membranes on either side of the cleft.

The synapses of Figs. 1-4B and 1-5 give good pictures of the structural basis of the chemical transmitter mechanism, which works just as described in the preceding chapter. An impulse propagates into the synaptic knob and liberates the transmitter contained in the vesicles. But it so happens that numerically the situation is very different. Accurate quantal studies have been done on these excitatory synapses on motoneurons by Kuno, exactly as was done on the neuromuscular synapse in the discovery of the number of vesicles or quanta of transmitter liberated by an impulse. The average quantal number comes out at only about 1, which is in contrast to the 100 to 200 at the neuromuscular synapse, as described in Chap. 2. This average quantal number per synapse is low because on the nerve cell are the many synapses from converging pathways, and there is very efficient summation of the individual excitatory synaptic actions, as indicated in Fig. 3-2J to M.

Just as with the neuromuscular synapse it can be assumed that, after the vesicles discharge their contained transmitter, they are refilled for further usage. The very narrow synaptic cleft in Figs. 1-4B and 1-5 is only about 200 to 300 Å across; nevertheless it is essential for the operation of the synapse. When a vesicle liberates its transmitter into the cleft, and so onto the postsynaptic membrane, this membrane has ionic gates opened with a consequent ionic flux across it. Synaptic transmission is effective only if extracellular current can flow along the synaptic cleft and so to extrasynaptic regions of the postsynaptic membrane, which are then depolarized (cf. Fig. 3-3A). Calculations on models of the synapse have shown that a cleft width of 200 to 300 Å is about optimal for the usual size of synapse—1 to 2 μm across. The synaptic knob must not be too far away else there will be inefficiency in the application of the transmitter to the postsynaptic membrane and an undue delay in operation due to diffusion time; and it cannot be too close else it will place too high a resistance on the flow of postsynaptic currents. It is of particular interest that the cleft is closed or almost so (the so-called gap junction) with synapses working by electrical transmission. As already mentioned, these synapses are not considered in this book because apparently they do not occur in the mammalian brain to any significant extent.

Figure 3-3*A* and *C* gives a summary of excitatory synaptic action. In *A* is a diagram of an excitatory synapse with the synaptic knob, and with the synaptic cleft enlarged by a factor of ten, as indicated by the scale. When an impulse reaches the synaptic knob, there is a quantal emission of transmitter, just as with the neuromuscular synapse. The transmitter has not yet been identified, but probably it is glutamate or a near relative. The transmitter acts on the postsynaptic membrane and causes current to flow inwards, as indicated, and thence in the circuit outwards from the membrane in general and in through the synaptic cleft. In this way the membrane is depolarized, just as with the endplate potential. In Fig. 3-3*C* the resting membrane potential is −70 mV. When the microelectrode is inserted across the membrane, the potential goes from 0 to −70 mV as indicated by the solid line and stays steady, just as in Fig. 1-11. Then the excitatory synaptic action causes the EPSP to rise up, as shown, so that it fires an impulse at a critical level of depolarization, as in Fig. 3-2*O* to *Q*.

But the question now is: What is the mechanism that is operated by the synaptic transmitter to cause the inward current flow across the postsynaptic membrane in *A*? It has been found that, if the membrane potential is displaced to a different level (Fig. 3-2*R*), as has been done with the endplate potential, the EPSP is progressively diminished to zero with decrease of the membrane potential from −70 to 0 mV and then reverses when the membrane potential is reversed. This is exactly what would happen if the EPSP were due to ionic diffusion. In Fig. 3-2*R* the reversal

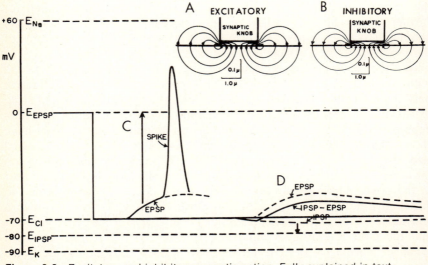

Figure 3-3 Excitatory and inhibitory synaptic action. Fully explained in text.

level is at about zero, i.e., the equilibrium potential for the ionic mechanism, E_{EPSP}, is zero, as shown in Fig. 3-3C. In reply to the question: What ionic gates are opened by this unknown transmitter? it can be said that on analogy with neuromuscular synapses it is believed to be both sodium gates and potassium gates. The E_{EPSP} would be a compromise value, as shown in Fig. 3-3C, between the equilibrium potentials for sodium, E_{Na} at +60 mV, and for potassium E_K at −90 mV (cf. Fig. 1-13).

In the normal operation of brain synapses, there is rarely a sharp single action by a synchronized volley of impulses, as in Fig. 3-2, but instead prolonged repetitive inputs. Hence, the question now arises: How effective is a long continued membrane depolarization in causing a prolonged impulse discharge? This question can be answered most directly by investigating the effects of steady depolarizing currents, instead of using synapses to fire a neuron. In Fig. 3-4A a microelectrode is inserted into a motoneuron and steady currents are passed to take charge off the surface membrane while at the same time the responses of the neuron are recorded. It is seen that a current of 7 nanoamperes (nA) just caused the neuron to fire, but the firing was slow and irregular. As the steady current was progressively increased, it produced more and more depolarization of the surface, and a faster and faster firing of the cell. Finally, with four times the threshold current, the neuron fired initially at the very high rate of at least 200 per second. In all cases the initial frequency slowed during the steady current application; nevertheless this experiment on prolonged impulse discharge reveals the immense range in the responses of neurons. Continuous synaptic bombardment is active in the same way. There are many species of neurons in the central nervous system that can be driven by intense synaptic bombardment to fire at 500 to 1000 per second. This is evidence of real synaptic power, and these neurons correspondingly exert strong synaptic power at their synapses.

In Fig. 3-4B a cell in the cerebral cortex is giving similar responses. The weakest current caused only one discharge. Again frequency of response increased sharply with intensity, and with a current just over four times threshold the initial frequency was over 200 per second.

It is immaterial whether depolarization is due to a steady synaptic bombardment or to an applied current. There is essentially the same response, depolarization generating impulse discharge, in a manner illustrating that intensity is coded by frequency, just as has been seen with receptor organs in Figs. 1-7 and 1-8A. The synapses and the neurons of the central nervous system are well adapted metabolically to respond continuously at frequencies as high as 100 per second and with peak responses as high as 500 per second. This is a performance far superior to that of neuromuscular synapses (cf. Fig. 2-8D and E). It used to be

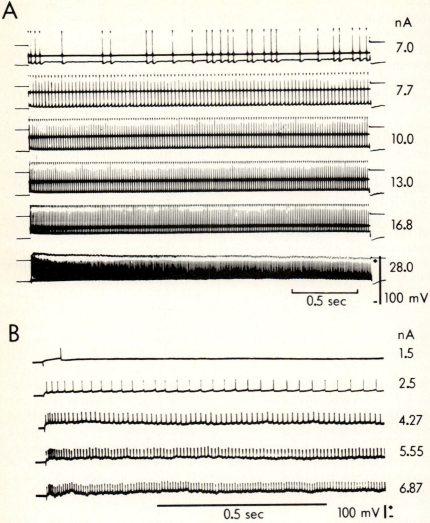

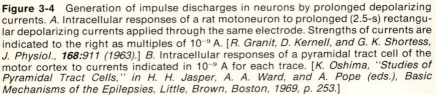

Figure 3-4 Generation of impulse discharges in neurons by prolonged depolarizing currents. *A.* Intracellular responses of a rat motoneuron to prolonged (2.5-s) rectangular depolarizing currents applied through the same electrode. Strengths of currents are indicated to the right as multiples of 10^{-9} A. [*R. Granit, D. Kernell, and G. K. Shortess, J. Physiol., 168:911 (1963).*] *B.* Intracellular responses of a pyramidal tract cell of the motor cortex to currents indicated in 10^{-9} A for each trace. [*K. Oshima, "Studies of Pyramidal Tract Cells," in H. H. Jasper, A. A. Ward, and A. Pope (eds.), Basic Mechanisms of the Epilepsies, Little, Brown, Boston, 1969, p. 253.*]

thought that one of the distinguishing properties of synapses was fatigue, but this is belied by the performance of synaptic mechanisms in the normal functioning of the brain.

Figure 3-5 gives a diagrammatic illustration of the manner in which coding of intensity by frequency is transformed at a synaptic relay by the cumulative depolarization due to EPSPs, and this in turn is again coded in frequency of discharge. For example, in stage A an assumed intensity-time course for stretch of a muscle gives the discharge of group Ia impulses in B and this in turn generates on a motoneuron the summed EPSPs (C). It is further assumed that there will be much the same bombardment of this motoneuron by impulses in several other group Ia afferent fibers that converge upon it, thus giving the aggregate EPSPs of D, which in its intensity-time course bears a not-seriously distorted resemblance of A. If D is sufficiently intense, it will in turn generate discharges of the motoneuron as shown in E, and these in turn the contraction, F, of the muscle, which in its intensity-time course is appropriately related to the stretch (A) which evoked it.

The significance of the transmutation from intensity to frequency and

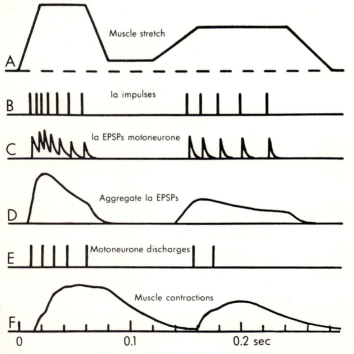

Figure 3-5   Transformations of intensity and frequency in the simplest reflex pathway. (*From Eccles, 1953.*)

vice versa can be appreciated only when account is taken of the integrative function of the nervous system. The most elementary level of integration is illustrated in Fig. 3-5, where stage *D* was derived from *C* by summation of the EPSPs produced by impulses converging from several different receptors. In this way intensity is transmitted by spatial as well as by temporal summation. Progressive increase in the intensity of a given stimulus will not only increase the frequency of discharge of a single receptor organ, as in Fig. 1-7, but also will cause other receptors to discharge and will increase the frequency of their discharge.

SYNAPTIC INHIBITORY ACTION

Figure 3-1*A* shows that the simplest inhibitory pathway in the spinal cord goes via a type of neuron that is specialized to exert an inhibitory synaptic action and nothing else. In 1946 Lloyd discovered that the Ia afferent fibers of a muscle inhibited motoneurons of the antagonist muscle. But the mechanism of this action was not known, nor was the inhibitory pathway diagrammed as in Fig. 3-1*A*. I had developed an electrical theory of inhibitory synaptic action, and eventually in 1951 my colleagues and I tested the theory by inserting a microelectrode inside the motoneuron (Fig. 3-1*B*) in order to see what inhibition did to the membrane potential. The electrical theory was proved wrong by our discovery that the inhibitory synapses produced a generalized increase of charge on the neuronal membrane, an effect called *hyperpolarization*.

In Fig. 3-6*A* to *C* there was graded stimulation of the group Ia fibers of the nerve to the antagonistic muscle (cf. Fig. 3-1*A*); the upper traces show the action potential of these fibers just as in Fig. 3-2*A* to *I*. There was an associated gradation of the inhibitory hyperpolarization of the membrane in the lower traces. This hyperpolarization we termed the *inhibitory postsynaptic potential, IPSP.* Its size is dependent upon the number of converging inhibitory synapses, just as with the excitatory synapses and the EPSPs in Fig. 3-2*A* to *F*. Figure 3-6*D* and *E* shows that the EPSP and IPSP of the same motoneuron are nearly mirror images. In both cases there is a brief flow of synaptic current for about 1 ms that effects the membrane potential change. Subsequently the membrane potential is restored to the initial level by ionic fluxes across the motoneuronal membrane in general (cf. Fig. 1-13*B*). This explains the similarity in time courses of the EPSP and IPSP. It is also a regular feature that the IPSP has a central latency about 1 ms longer than the EPSP, which is the time for traversing the inhibitory interneuron that is interpolated on the pathway (cf. Fig. 3-1*A*).

The inhibitory action of Ia impulses from a muscle on the motoneuron of an antagonist muscle was the first example of an inhibitory

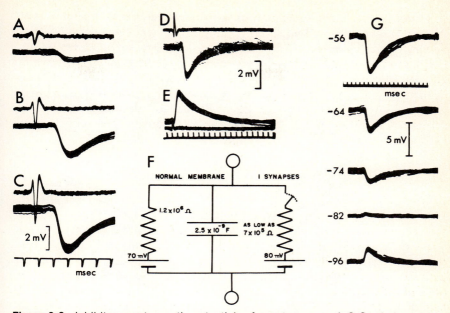

Figure 3-6 Inhibitory postsynaptic potentials of a motoneuron. *A-C.* Graded responses as described in the text. *D,E.* Comparison of EPSP and IPSP (time below *E* in
milliseconds). [*D. R. Curtis and J. C. Eccles, J. Physiol., 145:529 (1959).*] *F.* To the left
there is the formal electrical diagram of the membrane of a motoneuron (cf. Fig.
1-13*B*), while to the right the mode of operation of inhibitory synapses is symbolized by
the closing of the switch. *G.* Resembles Fig. 3-2*R* in showing effect of varying
membrane potential on the IPSP. [*J. S. Coombs, J. C. Eccles, and P. Fatt, J. Physiol.,
130:326 (1955).*]

mechanism studied by intracellular recording in the central nervous
system. It has turned out that the same general principles obtain for
almost all inhibitory actions in the brain, with the exception of presynaptic inhibition [to be discussed later (cf. Fig. 3-12)]. The techniques used in
the spinal cord have been applied at all levels of the central nervous
system. In many laboratories there is now a great ongoing enterprise of
identifying the excitatory and the inhibitory neurons in all the regions of
the brain, and of determining the manner of their interaction in complex
circuits. We have to discover at all these levels not only the neuronal
pathways but also the mechanisms at all synaptic relays, in particular the
synaptic transmitter substances at these relays and the ionic gates that
cause the different postsynaptic actions and so on. It is remarkable that
we are more advanced in answering these questions with respect to
inhibition than with excitation.

Figure 3-7 gives a kind of overall view of excitatory and inhibitory
synaptic action as we now understand it. In *C* the neuron is shown with an

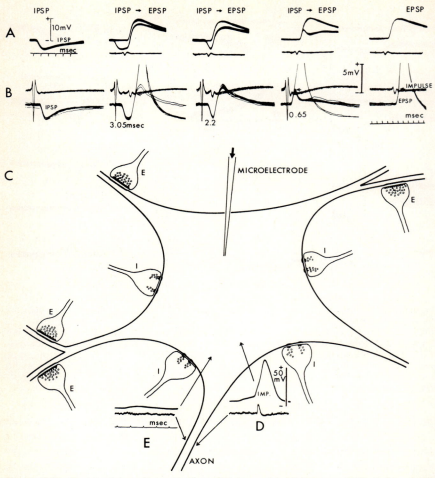

Figure 3-7 Summarizing diagram of excitatory and inhibitory synaptic action. In *C* the excitatory (E) and inhibitory (I) synapses are shown with characteristic histological features (cf. Fig. 1-4*B*). Full description in text.

intracellular microelectrode. It has been discovered that the excitatory synapses (E) tend to be out on the dendrites, as here drawn, while the inhibitory synapses (I) tend to be concentrated on the soma. Moreover there are structural differences, as already illustrated in the two synapses of Fig. 1-4*B* where, with glutaraldehyde fixation, the synaptic vesicles of the inhibitory synapse to the right have an ellipsoid configuration while in the excitatory to the left they are spherical. In addition, the membranes on either side of the synaptic cleft are less dense with inhibitory than with excitatory synapses. However, in essential structural features the two kinds of synapse are similar.

In Fig. 3-7*A* there are records of pure IPSPs and EPSPs. In the former, charge is put on the membrane, increasing the membrane potential from −70 to about −73 mV. The EPSP has an antagonistic action, decreasing the charge across the membrane. If you superimpose the IPSP on the EPSP, as in the fourth frame, the IPSP is seen to be very powerful in counteracting the EPSP, which is also shown alone in the same frame to aid comparison. In the third frame of Fig. 3-7*B* the IPSP very effectively suppresses the impulse discharge generated by the EPSP alone, which is illustrated in the last frame.

In Fig. 3-7*D* there is a good illustration of the EPSP generating an impulse discharge (cf. Fig. 3-2*O* to *Q*) that travels down the axon to be recorded as the brief spike in the lower trace. In *E* an initial inhibitory action reduces the EPSP so that it no longer generates an impulse, and the spike in the axon is also suppressed. Evidently inhibitory synapses achieve their effectiveness by generating the IPSP that directly counteracts the depolarizing action of the EPSPs. So we have the question: What are inhibitory synapses doing? solved at that level. There are, however, many more questions to answer.

We return now to Fig. 3-3*B*, where the inhibitory synaptic knob puts charge on the membrane via current going outwards across the subsynaptic membrane through the opened ionic gates. By the indicated lines of current flow, charge is increased across the neuronal membrane in general. We can now ask: What is the ionic mechanism responsible for the outward current across the subsynaptic membrane of the inhibitory synapse? A first step is to determine the equilibrium potential in the manner illustrated in Fig. 3-6*G*. The IPSP observed at the resting membrane potential (−74 mV) was increased by depolarizing the membrane (−64 mV and −56 mV) and was inverted by hyperpolarizing the membrane to −82 mV and still more at −96 mV. So in this way one can determine the point at which there is zero ionic flux during the IPSP. This is the equilibrium potential E_{IPSP} which is about −80 mV (Fig. 3-3*C* and *D*). The ionic gates are open but the ionic fluxes carry a zero net charge under these conditions.

We ask now: What are the ions? If you look at Fig. 3-3*C* and *D*, it seems likely that the ions are chloride and potassium. The equilibrium potential for the IPSP just balances at midway between the respective equilibrium potentials at approximately −70 mV for E_{Cl} and −90 mV for E_K. Since the equilibrium potential for sodium is as high as +60 mV, it is evident that even a minimal opening of sodium gates would displace the E_{IPSP} upwards, so preventing the hyperpolarizing action of the combined fluxes of K^+ and Cl^- ions. The role of Cl^- ions has been established by injecting Cl ions into the neuron and observing that the displacement of the E_{IPSP} is in accord with prediction, and is reversible.

Lux has presented evidence that there is an outward Cl^- pump across the neuronal membrane. As a consequence there could be a value for the Cl^- equilibrium potential of -80 mV and not at the resting membrane potential of -70 mV as in Fig. 1-13. Lux thus was able to explain the hyperpolarization of the IPSP as due solely to the opening of Cl^- gates, K^+ ions playing no significant role. However, my colleagues and I have recently found that Lux's experimental evidence with moto-neurons cannot be obtained even to the slightest extent with the very large IPSPs of the hippocampus (cf. Fig. 3-10A,B,C). With the hippocam-pal pyramidal cells there is no evidence for an outward Cl^-pump that is dependent on the internal concentratum of Cl^- as postulated by Lux; hence, the linked chloride-potassium ionic fluxes probably still obtain for the very important inhibitory synapses at higher levels of the brain.

Figure 3-8 gives models of inhibitory synaptic action. In A and B can be seen two ionic channels through the bimolecular leaflet of the surface membrane as illustrated in Fig. 1-12. One gate is closed and one opened by the steric actions of the transmitter molecule that has become attached to the receptor site. With inhibitory action in the mammalian central nervous system, it has been established that the inhibitory transmitters are amino acids, at some synapses *glycine* and at others *gamma aminobutyric acid* (GABA). It is further believed that these transmitters are packaged in the synaptic vesicles in inhibitory synaptic knobs (cf. Fig. 1-4B) and liberated into the synaptic cleft in a quantal manner. By diffusion a transmitter molecule would find a steric site as in Fig. 3-8B and so be able to pull the gate open for about 1 ms. Now K^+ and Cl^- ions can move by dif-fusion through the ionic channel so opened (Fig. 3-8D), and that gives the subsynaptic current that generates the inhibitory postsynaptic potential.

The ionic channels for inhibitory action seem to be lacking in chemical specificity. They merely have a size discrimination. For exam-ple, it has been shown that all 11 species of anions smaller than a critical size in the hydrated state (2.9 Å) will traverse the channels regardless of their chemical properties while all those larger than a critical size are excluded. Thus the activated inhibitory postsynaptic membrane acts merely as a sieve with a critical pore size, as is diagrammed in Fig. 3-8C. In D there is shown an electrical model incorporating the equilibrium potentials for the Cl^- and K^+ ions as given in Fig. 3-3C and the normal membrane model of Fig. 1-13B.

The ionic mechanism for generation of motoneuronal IPSPs accord-ing to the Lux hypothesis is illustrated in Fig. 3-8E and F, where the battery on the Cl^- channel in F is shown at -80 mV, in accord with the value postulated for E_{Cl} as a consequence of the outward Cl^-pump. The ionic channel is shown as being impermeable to K^+. Figure 3-8G and H shows in the same convention the mode of action of the presynaptic

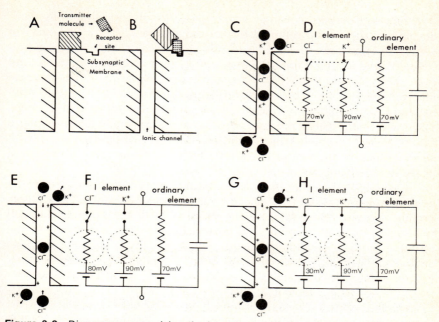

Figure 3-8 Diagrams summarizing the hypotheses relating to the ionic mechanisms employed by a variety of inhibitory synapses in producing IPSPs. Full description in text.

inhibitory transmitter (also GABA) in producing a depolarization (cf. Fig. 3-12). Further description will be given later. Not shown in Fig. 3-8 are many invertebrate inhibitory synapses where the opening of the ionic gates results in no change in the normal resting membrane potential. In the absence of a Cl⁻ pumping mechanism there is Cl⁻ equilibrium, but the inhibition is still effected because the depolarization of excitatory synapses is counteracted by the ionic mechanism that acts to hold the membrane potential at the resting level. It has been suggested that, if there are positive fixed charges on the channel, then the anions will go through and the cations will be repelled (Fig. 3-8*E* and *G*) and vice versa with fixed negative charges. This then is the general theory of inhibitory synaptic action. I think it is still too simple though it holds up remarkably well in a wide variety of tests.

GENERAL FEATURES OF SYNAPTIC TRANSMISSION IN THE BRAIN

Let us now return to the general diagram of chemical transmitting synapses in Fig. 2-11*A*. The wonderful biological process of evolution was not so uncompromisingly innovative. When good solutions were developed, they were retained by natural selection. They had survival value, and certainly chemical synaptic transmission had good survival value. It was invented long ago in relatively primitive invertebrates. And even the transmitter substances at mammalian synapses mostly have an invertebrate lineage. The detailed features of Fig. 2-11A apply to both excitatory and inhibitory synapses of the central nervous system (cf. Figs. 1-3B and 1-4B). There are the vesicles in the presynaptic terminals, a synaptic cleft of similar dimension, and a postsynaptic membrane with sensitivity to the transmitter substance that opens ionic gates, as indicated in the enlargement in Fig. 2-11B.

Essentially the same events occur with the excitatory synapses in the central nervous system as at the neuromuscular junction. The all-or-nothing impulse propagates to the terminal with the sodium Na_D and potassium K_D gates opening at a critical level of depolarization. At the terminal there is, in addition, opening of Ca_D gates so that calcium ions enter and participate in the process whereby the vesicles discharge their quantal content of transmitter into the synaptic cleft. This transmitter then diffuses to the subsynaptic membrane as in Fig. 2-10A and momentarily lodges on steric receptor sites (cf. Fig. 1-12) that allow it to open the sodium (Na_T) and potassium (K_T) gates that are shown in Fig. 2-11B. Unfortunately the excitatory transmitters at brain synapses are still largely unknown. It is acetylcholine in a few cases, but it could be glutamate or aspartate in many, and there probably are other substances such as the catecholamines.

The ionic fluxes through the Na_T and K_T channels depolarize the postsynaptic membrane enough to open the sodium and potassium gates concerned in impulse transmission, i.e., the Na_D and K_D gates shown in Fig. 2-11B open. The Na_D gates for impulse transmission in the brain are blocked in the same way by tetrodotoxin (TTX), and it is presumed that the potassium gates (K_D) are similarly blocked by intracellular tetraethylammonium (TEA). All evidence indicates that impulse transmission in the central nervous system is essentially the same as in peripheral nerves. Likewise it is assumed that the central depressant actions by manganese and magnesium are due to their effects in preventing Ca^{2+} ions moving in through the Ca_D channels.

With central inhibitory synapses the only difference is that the transmitters are the amino acids glycine or gamma aminobutyric acid (GABA), and that these transmitters open up channels across the subsynaptic membrane for chloride or for chloride and potassium, and strictly not for sodium. Nevertheless the essence of the story is the same. The presynaptic impulse opens the calcium gates at a certain level of depolarization, and the inward movement of Ca^{2+} ions liberates the transmitter quantally. The transmitter diffuses across the synaptic cleft and opens ionic gates with the consequent ionic fluxes that increase the charge across the subsynaptic membrane, so causing the flow of current (Fig. 3-3B) that hyperpolarizes the postsynaptic membrane.

SIMPLE NEURONAL PATHWAYS IN THE BRAIN

We now come to the neuronal pathways in the brain. There are many questions to be answered. How are the properties of individual synaptic actions effective in the linking of neuronal assemblages into some meaningful performance? What principles of neuronal organization can we define? How is information from receptor organs transmitted up to higher centers of the brain? In Chap. 4 we will treat the complementary problem of how the higher centers of the brain act on lower centers eventually to bring about motoneuronal discharge and so movement.

The Pathways for Ia Impulses

Figure 3-1A is a very simple pathway, where an Ia afferent fiber from a muscle enters the spinal cord and branches so that the discharges of this annulospiral receptor organ can exert both an excitatory and an inhibitory action. The inhibitory pathway has to be relayed through an interneuron because the afferent neuron itself can only act in an excitatory manner, presumably because it can only make the excitatory transmitter substance. So the transformation comes via an interneuron that has a different biochemical competence to make a different transmitter that has an inhibitory synaptic action. One can assume that this inhibitory interneuron has a genetic coding specified for this purpose and that this dates back to its origin in a differentiating mitosis, as will be discussed in Chap. 5. So far as we know, all afferent fibers entering the spinal cord are excitatory in their action. For central inhibitory action to occur there must be the transformation via interneurons specialized for inhibition, as shown for the Ia input in Fig. 3-1A. This requirement explains many of the design features in the brain. Figure 3-1A is an example of the simplest pathway producing excitation and reciprocal inhibition via a feed-forward inhibitory pathway.

The Renshaw Cell Pathway

In Fig. 3-9 there is a simple example of a feedback inhibitory pathway. In A a motoneuron is shown with its axon going all the way out to the muscle, as has already been illustrated in Fig. 2-1, and it acts there by the transmitter acetylcholine. The broken lines of the axon signify that it goes many centimeters after it leaves the spinal cord and before it reaches the muscle. But in the spinal cord this motoneuronal axon sends off collateral branches that make synapses on special neurons, *Renshaw cells,* as I called them after Birdsey Renshaw, a distinguished American neurobiologist who died from polio when he was very young. He discovered these cells and recorded their unique responses, but he did not live long enough to work out their mode of operation. It was the good fortune of my colleagues Fatt and Koketsu and myself to be able to pick up the story later and to give his name to this remarkable species of neuron.

Unfortunately the very existence of these neurons has been denied. These are neurons with a most interesting and beautiful performance, yet they have been demoted and denied neuronal status by inventing for them the absurd name Renshaw elements, which were assumed to be no more than the motor axon collaterals that were supposed to synapse directly on motoneurons! I am happy to say that a few years ago all of this opposition was effectively quelled. Jankowska in Sweden and Voorhoeve in Amsterdam and their associates have inserted into these cells fine micropipettes filled with procion yellow. First they established by electrical recording that the micropipette was in a Renshaw cell, then they squirted in the yellow dye, which spread through the whole branching structure of the cell so revealing in histological preparations the soma, dendrites, and axon, just as we had drawn them all along on the basis of our electrophysiological analyses.

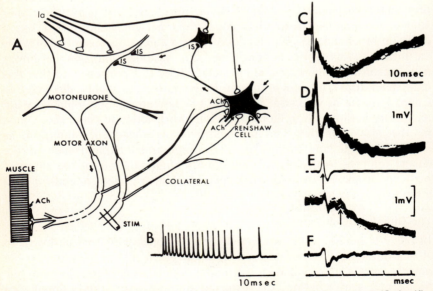

Figure 3-9 Feedback inhibition via Renshaw cells. Full description in text. IS signifies inhibitory synapses and ACh excitatory synapses operating with acetylcholine as transmitter. [*J. C. Eccles, P. Fatt, and K. Koketsu, J. Physiol., 126:524 (1954).*]

When, by electrical stimulation, impulses are set up in the motor axons, the Renshaw cells fire with a long burst, often at extremely high frequency, as in Fig. 3-9*B*. All kinds of pharmacological tests have established that the excitatory transmitter is acetylcholine, which is the same as at the neuromuscular synapses that are made by these same motor axons. This is in precise accord with Dale's principle, which I define as stating that at all the synapses formed by a neuron there is the same transmitter. For example, all synapses made by a motoneuron have acetylcholine as the transmitter despite great differences in the location (central or peripheral), in the mode of termination, and in the target cells. The Renshaw cell sends its axon to form inhibitory synapses on motoneurons. Figure 3-9*C* and *D* shows the large IPSP (at two different sweep speeds) produced in the motoneuron by the rapid Renshaw cell discharge (*B*). The latent period for the IPSP is shown by comparison of the extracellular record of the motoneuron (*F*) with the intracellular (lower trace of *E*), the IPSP being thus shown to begin at the arrow, which is only 1.1 ms after the volley in the motor axons—the arrow in the upper trace of *E* (note the faster time scale for *E* and *F*). This latency shows that there is just time for the pathway via Renshaw cells to the motoneuron that is drawn in Fig. 3-9*A*.

Furthermore, the Renshaw cell is seen in *A* also to give inhibitory synapses to an inhibitory interneuron. It so happens that in many cases this is the same inhibitory interneuron that is on the Ia inhibitory pathway to motoneurons (Fig. 3-1*A*). The action of the Renshaw cell on this inhibitory interneuron is to effect an inhibition of its inhibitory action, i.e., to diminish its inhibitory action, which is the equivalent of excitation. Removal of inhibition thus causes excitation by a process that is called *disinhibition*.

There is a lot of nice tricky physiology in this circuitry, but I want to concentrate on the feedback operation. What is the point of it? The more intensely this motoneuron in Fig. 3-9*A* fires impulses, the more it turns itself off by negative feedback via the Renshaw cells. You might well say: this is an example of poor design and is wasteful of neuronal activity. But it is not to be understood simply in the oversimplified diagram of Fig. 3-9*A*. Motoneurons activate many Renshaw cells via their axon collaterals, and each of these Renshaw cells inhibits many motoneurons. It is a very good example of the principles of divergence and of convergence mentioned earlier in this chapter. Any one Renshaw cell will be inhibiting an array of motoneurons largely regardless of function. When one group of motoneurons is firing strongly, it will exert a strong feedback inhibition via Renshaw cells on the whole ensemble of motoneurons in their neighborhood no matter what they are doing. As a consequence there is suppression of all weak discharges. Only the strongly excited neurons survive this inhibitory barrage. In this way the actual motor performance is made much more selective by the negative feedback eliminating the stray weakly responding motoneurons that would frequently cause some disorder in the movement.

The Hippocampal Basket Cell Pathway

Figure 3-10 is another example of a feedback pathway to a pyramidal cell in the hippocampus, which is a primitive part of the cerebral cortex. The neuron labeled p in *F* is the same kind of neuron as that in Fig. 1-3*B*, but it is shown inversely with its apical dendrite pointing downwards and its axon upwards. From the axon there is a collateral just like that of the motoneuron in Fig. 3-9*A*, and it makes an excitatory synapse on a neuron (b) that we can liken to a Renshaw cell because its axon (ba) branches profusely to give inhibitory synapses on the somata of this and adjacent pyramidal cells. This is another example of feedback inhibition. The more this pyramidal cell fires, the more it activates the feedback inhibition.

These inhibitory neurons (b) were called basket cells by Ramón y Cajal because of the basket-like embracement of the somata of the

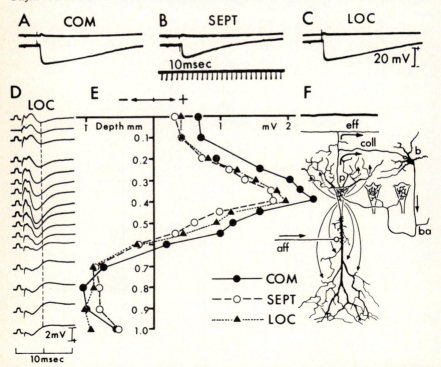

Figure 3-10 Feedback inhibition via basket cells in the hippocampus. Full description in text. [*P. Andersen, J. C. Eccles, and Y. Loyning, J. Neurophysiol., **27**:592, 608 (1964).*]

pyramidal cells. He thought they were excitatory, but in 1963, following earlier investigations by Spencer and Kandel, my colleagues and I established that they were inhibitory by a series of tests that are partly illustrated in Fig. 3-10. The very large IPSPs produced in a hippocampal pyramidal cell by the basket-cell synapses can be seen in the lower traces, *A, B,* and *C,* the upper traces being the control recordings just outside the cell. COM, SEPT, and LOC signify three different locations of stimulation for exciting the basket cells. Extracellular recording at the indicated depths gives the field potential profile in *D* and *E,* which indicates that the IPSP is generated at the level of the somata. The plottings in *E* show the field potentials recorded (*D*) at the depths corresponding to the drawing of the pyramidal cell in *F* and measured at the time of the vertical broken line in *D.* The maximum positivities occur at the depth of the somata in *F,* which indicates that the inhibitory synapses are located there. Reference to Fig. 3-3*B* reveals that the inhibitory synaptic site is the source of current flow to the rest of the cell, as shown by the arrows in Fig. 3-10*F.*

In this way it was established that the basket cells of Ramón y Cajal were inhibitory, and hence the location of inhibitory synapses was defined for the first time (Fig. 3-10*F*). Their clustered position on the soma of the hippocampal pyramidal cell is strategically an excellent place because their function is to stop the cell firing. This location on the soma provided the opportunity to identify inhibitory synapses in electron micrographs and to define their morphology, as has already been shown in Fig. 1-3*B* (e, f, g).

It has also been shown by Andersen and his associates that the numerous spine synapses on the dendrites, types *a* to *d* in Fig. 1-3*B,* are excitatory. These synapses are very powerful and can generate the discharge of impulses that propagate down the apical dendrite and so over the soma and down the axon. However the inhibitory synapses are also very powerful, as may be seen in the large IPSPs of Fig. 3-10*A* to *C.* Their location on the soma at the axonal origin gives them the final say as to whether the impulse be allowed to propagate down the axon. That is good strategical design to have the inhibitory synapses located at the optimal site. If, for example, they were located on the dendrites, impulses generated nearer to the soma would be able to fire down the axon without effective inhibitory constraint. With rare exceptions inhibitory synapses in all species of neurons are located on or close to the somata.

Generalizations on Inhibitory Pathways

In Fig. 3-11*A* there is a general diagram of the feedback pathways whose operations were illustrated in Figs. 3-9 and 3-10. In Fig. 3-11*B* there is the feed-forward pathway that has been illustrated for the Ia afferent fibers from muscle receptors (Fig. 3-1*A*), where collateral branches of the excitatory afferent fibers excite inhibitory interneurons that inhibit neurons in the forward direction. Both of these inhibitory pathways are now known not just to have a general value in keeping down the level of excitation and so suppressing discharges from all weakly excited neurons. In addition, they participate very effectively in neuronal integration, molding and modifying the patterns of neuronal responses. I always think that inhibition is a sculpturing process. The inhibition, as it were, chisels away at the diffuse and rather amorphous mass of excitatory action and gives a more specific form to the neuronal performance at every stage of synaptic relay. This suppressing action of inhibition can be recognized very clearly at higher levels of the brain—particularly in the cerebellum, as we shall see in Chap. 4.

The other point that I wish to emphasize is that inhibitory cells are uniquely specified neurons, as has already been stated. They act via unique transmitter substances, which in the spinal cord is almost always glycine while at the supraspinal levels, in the higher levels of the brain, it is almost always gamma aminobutyric acid (GABA). These two transmitters are very similar in their action, opening the same ionic gates, i.e., the gates for potassium and chloride ions, as in Fig. 3-8C and D. It would be expected that substances which interfere with inhibitory synaptic action would cause unfettered excitatory action of neuron onto neuron and so lead to convulsions. This is indeed the case. In fact, as shown by Curtis and his associates, there are two classes of convulsants, those like strychnine that selectively block glycine transmission, and those like bicuculline and picrotoxin that selectively block GABA transmission.

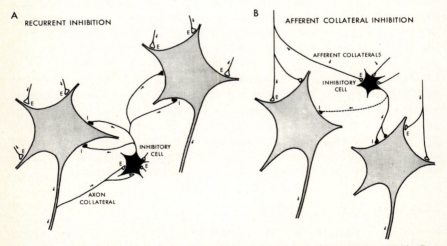

Figure 3-11   The two types of inhibitory pathways, feedback in *A*, feed-forward in *B*, as described in text.

The unfolding of the central inhibitory story of the brain has been a great success, and it is now better understood that the central excitatory story. At least 10 supraspinal inhibitory pathways are now known to work by GABA and in almost as many spinal pathways the transmitter is shown to be glycine. A very important generalization is that neurons of the mammalian brain are either excitatory or inhibitory—never both. My colleagues and I first published this postulate in 1954. It has been attacked very heavily since. Initially we had only four species of inhibitory neurons as the basis of that generalization; nevertheless it seemed that it should be so because of the uniqueness of the inhibitory chemical transmitter operations and of the specific antagonism by strychnine. It was related to Dale's principle, because inhibitory synaptic action should be effected by transmitter substances specified for the purpose. Now it is possible to enumerate over 30 species of inhibitory neurons in different parts of the mammalian brain that are doing nothing else but inhibition, working presumably by either GABA or glycine. Likewise an even larger number of species of pure excitatory neurons have been identified. There are no known ambivalent neurons in the mammalian brain. In attempts to unravel the neuronal pathways in the brain it is a great help to recognize that the first big step is to identify the excitatory and inhibitory neurons. This criterion of a sharp classification is of essential importance in trying to discover the mode of operation of cell assemblages in the nuclear and cortical structures of the brain. In the first instance you don't have to bother about asking the more confusing question: Are some species of neurons both inhibitory and excitatory? However, the possibility of exceptional neuronal operation has always to be kept in mind. We now come to the nearest approach to such an exception. It occurs in the special synaptic mechanisms giving what is called presynaptic inhibition.

PRESYNAPTIC INHIBITION

The inventiveness of the evolutionary process is well illustrated by a quite different neuronal mechanism for depressing synaptic excitatory action. As its name signifies, in *presynaptic inhibition* the inhibitory action is effected by depressing the output of excitatory transmitter by the presynaptic terminals and not by antagonizing the postsynaptic action of that transmitter as in Fig. 3-7A and B, for example. Presynaptic inhibition is very widespread and powerful at lower levels of the brain. It is best studied on primary afferent fibers at their synaptic relays in the spinal cord, as diagrammed in Figs. 1-6 and 3-1A, or at their relays in the *dorsal column nuclei* as in Fig. 3-13 (cuneate nuc.). All impulses in large afferent fibers exert a presynaptic inhibitory action on the central terminals of afferent fibers.

Figure 3-12 is a composite picture illustrating the basic synaptic structure and mode of action in presynaptic inhibition. As already mentioned in relation to Fig. 1-4A, synaptic endings are observed to occur on presynaptic terminal fibers as shown in Fig. 3-12. These axo-axonic synapses are made by *presynaptic inhibitory fibers* that are the axonal branches of special interneurons in the spinal cord. Thus the pathway is via interneurons just as for postsynaptic inhibition (cf. Fig. 3-1A), but it is by different interneurons.

Presynaptic inhibition is explained by the following sequence of events. Impulses on the presynaptic inhibitory fiber depolarize the presynaptic terminal, as can be seen in the intracellular recordings from it in Fig. 3-12C, for one, two, or four stimuli to the presynaptic inhibitory input. As a consequence of this depolarization, the action potential of impulses in the presynaptic terminal is diminished in size, which entails a depression of output of transmitter, just as has been observed for peripheral synapses (cf. Fig. 2-13), and that is demonstrated by the diminished EPSPs in Fig. 3-12A and B when compared to the controls (Con). This diminution accounts for the inhibitory depression of the reflex discharge evoked by the synaptic excitation. For example, in Fig. 3-12D the second and third traces show the reflex inhibition at different test intervals and the first trace is the control reflex.

It is important to distinguish sharply between the modes of operation of presynaptic and postsynaptic inhibition. In presynaptic inhibition excitatory transmitter output is reduced and the electrical properties of the postsynaptic membrane are unaffected (as indicated by the unchanged potentials produced by square pulses in Fig. 3-12F and G relative to the control in E) whereas the EPSPs below show the effectiveness of the presynaptic inhibition. In postsynaptic inhibition the presynaptic terminals are unaffected; the inhibitory action is exerted solely on the postsynaptic membrane which is hyperpolarized (Figs. 3-6 and 3-7). It remains to issue a warning against the attempts still being made to attribute presynaptic inhibition to postsynaptic inhibitory action far out on the neuronal dendrites—the so-called "remote inhibition." Another confusion arises from attempts to account for the presynaptic inhibitory effect by the extracellular accumulation of potassium that does, of course, occur with intense neuronal activity.

There is now good evidence that the presynaptic inhibitory transmitter is GABA. GABA resembles presynaptic inhibitory synapses in producing a depolarization of the presynaptic terminals of primary afferent fibers. Both actions (either of GABA or the presynaptic synapses) are selectively depressed by bicuculline and picrotoxin. Furthermore, GABA effects the depolarization of the presynaptic terminals largely by opening Cl^- gates (Nicoll, Nishi) as indicated in Fig. 3-8G and H. The

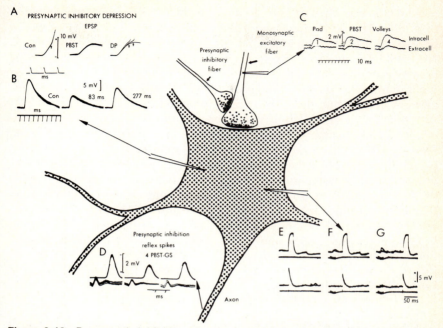

Figure 3-12 Presynaptic inhibition, structures, and various types of responses associated therewith. Full discussion in text. *A* shows the effect of a brief repetitive stimulation of the presynaptic inhibitory fibers of two muscle nerves (PBST and DP) in reducing the size of a monosynaptic EPSP below the control level (Con). In *B* there is a much greater reduction of the EPSP at the indicated times after a prolonged presynaptic inhibitory activation. [*J. C. Eccles, Progr. Brain Res.,* **12**:65 *(1965)*.] *D* shows the diminution of monosynaptic reflex discharges from gastrocnemius motoneurons (see text). *E* to *G* are described in the text. [*From E. Eide, I. Jurna, and A. Lundberg, "Conductance Measurements from Monotneuones during Presynaptic Inhibition," in C. von Euler, S. Skoglund, and V. Soderberg (eds.), Structure and Function of Inhibitory Neuronal Mechanisms, Pergamon, New York, 1968, p. 215.*]

equilibrium potential for this ionic mechanism is about -30 mV, which indicates that there is an inward Cl^- pump in the presynaptic fibers that causes the E_{Cl} to be about 40 mV in the depolarizing direction from the resting membrane potential. In the frog this E_{Cl} value obtains even as far peripherally as the dorsal root ganglion cells. It is of interest that the transmitter, GABA, opens Cl^- gates in its action in both postsynaptic and presynaptic inhibition.

One generalization about presynaptic inhibition is that it has no patterned topography. It is widely dispersed over the afferents of a limb with but little tendency to focal application. For example, presynaptic inhibitory action by the afferent fibers of a muscle is effective on the afferents from all muscles of that limb regardless of function. It is not selective on one class of muscle, or on the muscles acting at any one joint of a limb. This widespread, nonspecific character is exactly what would be expected for the general suppressor influence of negative feedback. Nevertheless, there is organization or pattern in the distribution of presynaptic inhibition; this pattern depends on the class or modality of the afferent fiber on which the presynaptic inhibition falls, the cutaneous afferent fibers being the most strongly affected.

Another generalization is that presynaptic inhibition is much more effective at the primary afferent level than at the higher levels of the brain. However, it has been shown to exercise an important inhibitory influence on pathways through the thalamus and lateral geniculate body and it is utilized by descending pathways from the cerebrum for inhibitory action on synapses made by primary afferent fibers either in the spinal cord or in the dorsal column nuclei as in Fig. 3-13. So far there has been no evidence for presynaptic inhibition at the highest levels of the mammalian brain, i.e., the cerebellar cortex and the cerebral cortices—both the neocortex and the hippocampus. An interesting evolutionary problem is raised by this rejection of presynaptic inhibition at higher levels of the brain in favor of postsynaptic inhibition.

THE AFFERENT PATHWAY FOR CUTANEOUS SENSE

Figure 3-13 is a diagram of the simplest pathway from receptor organs in the skin up to the cerebral cortex. For example a touch on the skin causes a receptor to fire impulses as illustrated in Fig. 1-7A. These travel directly up the dorsal columns of the spinal cord (the cuneate tract for the hand and arm) and then after a synaptic relay in the cuneate nucleus and another one in the thalamus, the pathway reaches the cerebral cortex. There are only two synapses on the way and you might say, why have any at all? Why not have a direct line? The point is that each one of these relays gives an opportunity for an inhibitory action that sharpens the neuronal signals by eliminating all the weaker excitatory actions, such as would occur when the skin touches an ill-defined edge. In this way a much more sharply defined signal eventually comes up to the cortex and there again there is the same inhibitory sculpturing of the signal. As a consequence touch stimuli can be more precisely located and evaluated. In fact because of this inhibition a strong cutaneous stimulus is often surrounded by an area that has reduced sensitivity. Though not shown in the diagram there is presynaptic inhibition as well as postsynaptic inhibition in the thalamus.

Also shown in Fig. 3-13 are the pathways down from the cerebral cortex to both of these synaptic relays on the cutaneous pathway. In this way, by exerting presynaptic and postsynaptic inhibition, the cerebral

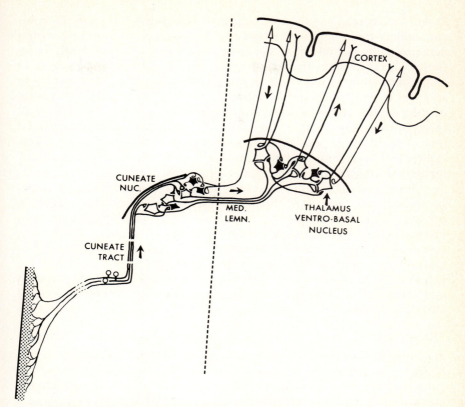

Figure 3-13 Pathway to the sensorimotor cortex for cutaneous fibers from the forelimb. Note the inhibitory cells shown in black in both the cuneate nucleus and the ventrobasal nucleus of the thalamus. The inhibitory pathway in the cuneate nucleus is of the feed-forward type and in the thalamus it is the feedback type. Also shown is one presynaptic inhibitory pathway to an excitatory synapse of a cuneate tract fiber. Efferent pathways from the sensorimotor cortex are shown exciting the thalamocortical relay cells and exciting both types of inhibitory neuron in the cuneate nucleus.

cortex is able to block these synapses and so protect itself from being bothered by cutaneous stimuli that can be neglected. This is of course what happens when you are very intensely occupied, for example, in carrying out some action or in experiencing or in thinking. Under such situations you can be oblivious even of severe stimulation. For example, in the heat of combat severe injuries may be ignored. At a less severe level it has long been a practice to give counterirritation to relieve pain. Presumably in this way there is produced inhibitory suppression of the pain pathway to the brain. If I were to give an explanation of acupuncture, it would be in similar terms. The needle stimuli cause stimulation of cutaneous pathways that depress the pain pathways by inhibitory action at the various relays to the cortex, just as with counterirritation. Then we can explain the afferent anesthesias of hypnosis or of Yoga also by the cerebral pathways inhibiting the cutaneous pathways to the brain. In all these cases discharges from the cerebral cortex down the pyramidal tract and other pathways will exert an inhibitory blockage at the relays in the spinocortical pathways such as those diagrammed in Fig. 3-13. This ability of the cerebral cortex is important because it is undesirable to have all receptor organ discharges from your body pouring into your brain all the time. The design pattern of successive synaptic relays each with various central and peripheral inhibitory inputs gives opportunity for turning off inputs according to the exigencies of situations.

Figure 1-7A illustrates the firing of one of those cutaneous receptors in response to graduated pressure giving the indentations listed in microns. Within limits the more the indentation the faster the firing rate. It is a very good example of intensity being coded by frequency. This same coding is operative all along the pathway to the cerebral cortex, which in this way receives the coded signals. Figure 3-14 is a diagram of the cerebral cortex showing two afferent fibers coming up from the thalamus and then relaying through excitatory and inhibitory neurons (E and I stellate cells) so that both inhibitory and excitatory action is exerted on the pyramidal cells.

But Fig. 3-14 is a greatly simplified picture of the real state of affairs. An important design feature of the cerebral cortex is that the whole neuronal machinery activated by many similar fibers of some specific cutaneous input is arranged in a column that is vertically oriented to the cortical surface, as will be further discussed in relation to Fig. 4-6. So, as a first approximation, we can say that all these neurons in Fig. 3-14 are engaged in an integrated operation. The same kind of cutaneous sense (modality) from the cutaneous area provides the input to a column, where there is mutual help in neuronal activation. You might ask, what is the point of this columnar arrangement? Isn't it enough for each afferent fiber to register its own ongoing activity in isolation? The point is that impulses in one fiber and discharges from one neuron or a few neurons will be virtually ineffective at the next stage of the synaptic relay. There must be many parallel lines because the input from one afferent fiber is lost in all the incessant "noise" of background firing, which is the actual state of the neurons of a "resting" cerebral cortex (cf. Figs. 4-4B and 6-5A). But, if you have 100 or even perhaps 20 fibers coming in with approximately synchronized bursts of impulses, the whole ensemble of cells in the column would be stirred up in a highly significant manner. This in turn will result in a spreading of meaningful signals widely and selectively in the cerebral cortex that could lead eventually to a conscious experience, as will be discussed in Chap. 6.

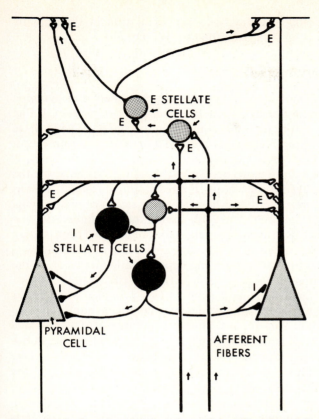

Figure 3-14 Postulated connections of specific afferent fibers (cf. Fig. 3-13) to the neocortical pyramidal cells. Note that the inhibitory path is through inhibitory cells that are activated either directly by the afferent fibers or by mediation of excitatory interneurons. Also note the various degrees of complexity of the excitatory pathways to the pyramidal cells. Arrows indicate direction of impulse propagation.

In the next chapter (Fig. 4-5) the columnar arrangement in the cerebral cortex will be shown to have a further function in that it provides a discriminatory judgment. The inhibitory neurons in any column tend to have their axons distributed not in the column as is shown in Fig. 3-14 but laterally thereto (Fig. 4-6). In this way activation of any column initiates inhibition in the immediately surrounding cortex, and this of course is a reciprocal phenomenon. It is again an example of integration by conflict. The most intense inputs achieve recognition by their effectiveness in suppressing the weaker inputs in their surround. This surround inhibition also serves to sharpen the cerebral patterns evoked by inputs. For example, such a sharpening enhances the ability to distinguish between two cutaneous stimuli very close together, the so-called two-point discrimination. The topology of the body representation in the somatic afferent pathway has been well described by Werner.

INHIBITION BY RECIPROCAL SYNAPSES

In the schematized diagrams of Fig. 3-11 it is assumed that synaptic excitation of the inhibitory neurons generates impulse discharges (cf. Fig. 3-9B) and that the inhibitory action is consequent on the passage of these impulses to the inhibitory synapses and the liberation of transmitter therefrom, in the manner that has been described in detail in Chap. 2. However, it was shown there that a presynaptic impulse was not essential for the liberation of transmitter from a presynaptic terminal. It was sufficient merely to produce an equivalent depolarization of the terminal by an applied current (Figs. 2-8C and 2-12) so that the Ca_D gates would be opened and the quanta of transmitter released. It has now been shown that in certain inhibitory neurons the liberation of transmitter similarly is produced by an electrotonically spreading depolarization and not by the depolarization of an impulse.

Rall, Shepherd, and their colleagues have provided convincing evidence, both histological and physiological, that this synaptic mechanism plays as important role on the olfactory pathway from the smell receptors to the brain, which is diagrammed in Fig. 3-15. In A the mitral cells (m) on the pathway have large secondary dendrites (SD) that make synapses with gemmules on the strange dendrite-like branches of the inhibitory granule cells (g). When examined by electron microscopy these synapses show a reciprocal structure as shown in B, which represents an enlargement of one gemmule synapse. The mitral dendrite (SD) is presynaptic to the gemmule in the synapse (E) to the left in B, which has a typical excitatory synaptic structure (cf. Fig. 1-4B to the left). On the other hand to the right in B, in the synapse (I), the mitral dendrite is postsynaptic to the gemmule and it displays a typical inhibitory-type synapse (cf. Fig. 1-4B, to the right).

The mode of operation of this reciprocal synaptic arrangement is shown by the current flow diagram drawn as in Fig. 3-3A and B. Depolarization of the secondary dendrite by an impulse in the mitral cell (m) causes the output of excitatory transmitter and depolarization of the gemmule in the ordinary manner of excitatory synaptic action, as shown for the synapse to the left in B. This depolarization of the gemmule is sufficient for the activation of its inhibitory synapse I on the secondary dendrite without the intervention of an impulse. There is a consequent flow of current hyperpolarizing this dendrite in the manner of Fig. 3-3B. Thus the proposed inhibitory pathway from mitral cell to mitral cell is by a very short linkage through the inhibitory granule cells, which may even

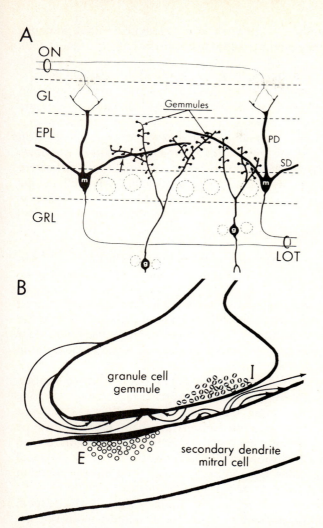

Figure 3-15   Reciprocal synapses in olfactory bulb. *A.* Layers and connections in the olfactory bulb. (*Adapted from Ramon y Cajal, Histologie du Systeme Nerveux, 1911.*) GL, glomerular layer; EPL, external plexiform layer; GRL, granular layer; ON, olfactory nerve; LOT, lateral olfactory tract; g, granule cell; m, mitral cell; PD, primary mitral dendrite; SD, secondary mitral dendrite. *B* shows diagrammatically the enlargement of the reciprocal synapse indicated by the arrow in *A.*

be within a single gemmule as in Fig. 3-15*B*. However, it is assumed that the electrotonic spread of depolarization in the granule cell dendrite is adequate for the depolarization of one gemmule to spread to others that in turn inhibit secondary dendrites, often from many mitral cells, as indicated in *A.* The physiological significance of this reciprocal synaptic mechanism can be understood when it is recognized that a dense meshwork is made by the gemmule-studded branches of the granule cells and by the secondary dendrites of mitral cells. It is thus possible for mitral cells very effectively to inhibit each other via the reciprocal synapses.

This remarkable new development gives an additional manner in which inhibitory interneurons can be effective in producing postsynaptic inhibition. Furthermore, Dowling and his colleagues have shown that similar reciprocal synapses occur with horizontal and amacrine cells in the retina, which likewise are inhibitory. There could be other examples of such reciprocal synapses in the cerebral cortical systems, where dendro-dendritic synapses were found to be numerous by Powell and his colleagues.

PRINCIPLES OF NEURONAL OPERATION

What can we now say as a result of this study of individual nerve cells in the brain and of some of the simplest organizations of them? There will be further examples in Chaps. 4 and 6. Can we define principles of operation? I think that our understanding of the brain has now advanced so far that we can enunciate a number of general principles in a quite dogmatic manner. I now proceed to do this seriatim because it will clear the way for advancing in our further attempts to understand the brain in the remaining three chapters.

First, in the brain all transmission at a distance is by the propagation of nerve impulses. These are the all-or-nothing messages that travel along fibers and which were the main theme of Chap. 1. There is a minor reservation with respect to synaptic actions at close range of the type illustrated in Fig. 3-15, where it can be by cable-like transmission. It is to be understood that this exclusion principle does not apply to the chemical transport of macromolecules along nerve fibers that will be considered in Chap. 5.

Second, we have the principle of divergence, as already defined. There are numerous branchings of all axons with a correspondingly great opportunity for wide dispersal because the impulses discharged by a neuron travel along all its axon branches to activate the synapses thereon. The divergence may be as low as 10, but values may be in the hundreds, as will be illustrated in Chap. 4.

Third, we have the complementary principle of convergence. All neurons receive synapses from many neurons, usually of several different species, as illustrated for the hippocampal pyramidal cell in Fig. 1-3*B*; also, they receive both excitatory and inhibitory synapses. It is doubtful if any neuron in the brain receives only excitation, and certainly there is no example of a purely inhibitory reception. The numbers of synapses on individual neurons are usually measured in hundreds or thousands, the highest recorded being around 80,000.

Fourth, there is the successive transmutation from electrical to chemical and back to electrical in each synaptic transfer. From this process there arises the integrational properties of the nervous system. There is the necessity for convergence of many synaptic excitations before a neuronal discharge is evoked, and there is further opportunity for synaptic inhibitory action to prevent this discharge. In Chap. 2 and the earlier part of Chap. 3, I concentrated on the principles of chemical synaptic transmission: the presynaptic impulse, the chemical transmitter substances, their quantal liberation by impulses, their action on the postsynaptic membrane opening ionic gates with the consequent transmutation to an electrical event. This is the basic principle of communication in the brain. I am stressing it because it is fashionable for psychologists these days to propose that there is another kind of communication by what they call "the slow potential microstructure." They endow these potential fields with integrative or synthetic properties in their own right, whereas we can with assurance ascribe their production to the flow of currents generated by synaptic action in the ordinary process of synaptic transmission, as diagrammed in Fig. 3-3*A* and *B*, and revealed in depth profile in the hippocampal cortex (Fig. 3-10*D* and *E*). There is no neurobiological evidence that these currents are anything more than a spin-off from chemical synaptic transmission. Doubtless, if large enough, electrical fields would slightly modify the production of impulse discharge by synaptic action. But this would be diffuse and carry no significant information. Neurophysiological investigations strongly emphasize the almost exclusive role of impulses in coding information transmission both in the peripheral nervous system and in the brain, intensity being coded by frequency of firing. Figure 3-15 illustrates the rare exceptions. Figure 3-5 gives a diagrammatic representation of a very simple example. But that principle can be extended indefinitely for sequence after sequence of synaptic transmission.

Fifth, in the brain there is almost always background firing of neurons. If there is coding by frequency of firing, then it has to be remembered that this coding is superimposed on a background of incessant, irregular discharge. Even when you are asleep the neurons of your cerebral cortex are firing impulses. Actually some fire even faster when you are asleep than when you are awake. The problem is to extract a reliable performance out of the nervous system, considering that it has so much background noise. This is done by having many lines in parallel, all carrying much the same signals. The columnar arrangement of input areas in the cerebrum (Figs. 4-5, 4-6, 6-5*B*) does just this, and there are other examples now being discovered where neurons of similar connectivities are arranged in clusters, as, for example, in the cerebellar cortex and nuclei (Chap. 4). The same kinds of neurons are organized together, receiving the same kinds of message on the whole and transmitting the same kind of coded output to another cluster of neurons. Because of the incessant background noise the responses of one neuron are lost. The neurons have to "shout together" as it were to get the message across and so make a reliable signal above all the background noise. This will be one of our problems in Chaps. 4 and 6, namely to see how signals are lifted out of noisy backgrounds by collusion of many cells lying together in clusters and working together in parallel.

Sixth, there is the whole question of inhibition coming in and sharpening signals and controling neuronal discharges by both the feedforward and feedback circuits that have been fully described in this chapter.

Seventh, I would stress that everything that goes on in your brain has a basis in neuronal events and can be measured in terms of signals which by synaptic operation fire neurons and so on in most complex organizational patterns. Chapter 4 will be an introduction to some attempts to illuminate some simpler levels that are concerned with the control of movement. We are attempting to understand some simpler levels—some of the simpler jigsaw components of the immense ensemble of complexity—and so gradually to understand more and more complex levels of brain action. Finally, in Chap. 6 we will be engaged on the most important and challenging problem of all, namely the events in the cerebral cortex, the highest level of the brain, which again have to be understood as the weaving by impulses of the complex spatiotemporal patterns that have been likened by Sherrington to the weaving of an enchanted loom. But again all we will postulate at the neuronal level is impulse transmission and the synaptic mechanisms responsible for the impulse discharges.

REFERENCES

Allen, G. I., J. C. Eccles, R. A. Nicoll, T. Oshima, and F. J. Rubia (1976): "The Ionic Mechanisms Concerned in Generating the IPSPs of Hippocampal Pyramidal Cells," *J. Physiol.*, (in press).

Curtis, D. R. (1969a): "The Pharmacology of Spinal Postsynaptic Inhibition," in K. Akert and P. G. Waser (eds.), *Progress in Brain Research*, vol. 31, Elsevier, Amsterdam, pp. 171–189.

Curtis, D. R. (1969b): "Central Synaptic Transmitters," in H. H. Jasper, A. A. Ward, and A. Pope (eds.), *Basic Mechanisms of the Epilepsies*, Little, Brown, Boston, pp. 105–129.

Curtis, D. R., and D. Felix (1971): "The Effect of Bicuculline upon Synaptic Inhibition in the Cerebral and Cerebellar Cortices of the Cat," *Brain Res.*, 34:301–321.

Eccles, J. C. (1957): *The Physiology of Nerve Cells*, The Johns Hopkins Press, Baltimore.

Eccles, J. C. (1964): *The Physiology of Synapses*, Springer, Berlin, Göttingen, and Heidelberg.

Eccles, J. C. (1965): "The Synapse," *Sci. Amer.*, 1965; reprinted in *Physiological Psychology*, Freeman, San Francisco, 1971, pp. 136–146.

Eccles, J. C. (1966): "The Ionic Mechanisms of Excitatory and Inhibitory Synaptic Action," *Ann. N.Y. Acad. Sci.*, 137:473–495.

Eccles, J. C. (1969a): "Excitatory and Inhibitory Mechanisms in the Brain," in H. H. Jasper, A. A. Ward, and A. Pope (eds.), *Basic Mechanisms of the Epilepsies*, Little, Brown, Boston, pp. 229–252.

Eccles, J. C. (1969b): *The Inhibitory Pathways of the Central Nervous System*, Sherrington Lectures, Liverpool University Press, Liverpool.

Granit, R. (1966): "Effects of Stretch and Contraction on the Membrane of Motoneurones," Nobel Symposium I, *Muscular Afferents and Motor Control*, Almqvist & Wiksells, Stockholm, pp. 37–50.

Gray, E. G. (1970): "The Fine Structure of Nerve," *Comp. Biochem. Physiol.*, 36:419–448.

Ito, M., (1976): "Roles of GABA Neurons in Integrated Functions of the Vertebrate CNS," in E. Roberts, T. W. Chase, and D. B. Tower (eds.), *GABA in Nervous System Function*, Raven, New York, pp. 427–448.

Krnjević, K. (1974): "Chemical Nature of Synaptic Transmission in Vertebrates," *Physiol. Rev.*, 54:418–540.

Kuno, M. (1971): "Quantum Aspects of Central and Ganglionic Synaptic Transmission in Vertebrates," *Physiol. Rev.*, 51:647–678.

Lux, H. D. (1971): "Ammonium and Chloride Extrusion: Hyperpolarizing Synaptic Inhibition in Spinal Motoneurones," *Science*, 173:555–557.

McLennan, H. (1969): *Synaptic Transmission*, Saunders, Philadelphia and London.

Mountcastle, V. B. (1966): "The Neural Replication of Sensory Events in the Somatic Afferent System," in J. C. Eccles (ed.), *Brain and Conscious Experience*, Springer, New York, pp. 85–115.

Mountcastle, V. B. (1975): "The View from Within: Pathways to the Study of Perception," *The Johns Hopkins Medical Journal*, 136:109–131.

Rall, W. (1970): "Dendritic Neuron Theory and Dendrodendritic Synapses in a Simple Cortical System," in F. O. Schmitt (ed.), *The Neurosciences*, Rockefeller University Press, New York, pp. 552–565.

Reese, T. S., and G. M. Shepherd (1972): "Dendro-dendritic Synapses in the Central Nervous System," in G. D. Pappas and D. P. Purpura (eds.), *The Structure and Function of Synapses*, Raven, New York, pp. 121–136.

Schmidt, R. F. (1971): "Presynaptic Inhibition in the Vertebrate Central Nervous System," *Ergebn. Physiol.*, 63:21–108.

Werner, G. (1970): "The Topology of the Body Representation in the Somatic Afferent Pathway," in F. O. Schmitt (ed.), *The Neurosciences*, Rockefeller University Press, New York, pp. 605–617.

The Control of Movement by the Brain

INTRODUCTION

In the first three chapters I have dealt with basic problems of neural communication: first, impulse transmission in nerve, the signal that runs along single nerve fibers; second, transmission at the simplest peripheral synapses, such as the neuromuscular junction, where a chemical transmission mediates between the impulse transmissions; and third, transmission at the simplest excitatory and inhibitory synapses in the central nervous system, from neuron to neuron. I have also dealt with the simplest pathways in the central nervous system, with reflexes, and with such elemental operations as facilitation and negative feedback. All of that is preliminary to the consideration of some meaningful reactions of the nervous system, which will be the theme of this chapter.

Most important problems arise in an attempt to give an account of how we can move. How can we control our musculature to give us actions in accordance with the situations that we find ourselves in? How can I, for example, move my arm so that with my eyes shut I can smoothly put my finger on the tip of my nose? But you all can think of much more complicated movements in the immense repertoire of skill that you have in games, in technology, in playing musical instruments, and most importantly and very complexly in speech and song and gesture, so that your whole personality can stand revealed. And it stands revealed simply because of your movement by your muscular contractions, as, for example, in all facial gesture and eye movement. If you are fixed like a corpse with a mask-like face, you reveal no personality, you are as good as dead!

MOTOR CONTROL FROM THE CEREBRAL CORTEX

The Motor Cortex

After this introduction it is appropriate that I begin with voluntary control, which is contrary to the usual convention, where a start is made with simple reflexes with a gradual ascent to the more complex. I want to deal firstly with voluntary control because I can in this way relate my story to your experiences. Figure 4-1 shows the position of the left motor cortex as a band across the surface of the cerebral hemisphere. It lies just anterior to the central fissure (the fissure of Rolando, f. Rol.), and many of its constituent nerve cells are pyramidal cells (cf. Fig. 1-2*B*) whose axons are in the nerve fibers running down the pyramidal tract. The *motor cortex* is a tremendously important structure, but it is not the prime initiator of a movement, such as a voluntary bending of your finger. It is only the final relay station of what has been going on in widely dispersed areas in your cerebral cortex, as will be illustrated in Fig. 4-3. The pyramidal cells of the motor cortex with their axons passing down the *pyramidal tract* are important because they provide a direct channel out from the brain to the motoneurons (Fig. 4-2) that in turn cause the muscle contractions as described in the earlier chapters and as illustrated in Fig. 2-1.

When brief stimulating currents are passed through electrodes placed on the surface of the motor cortex, there are contractions of localized groups of muscles. In this way it was discovered that all the various parts of the body are represented in a strip-like map that is shown in Fig. 4-1. This was done first with monkeys and anthropoid apes, but the map has now been completely established for humans, particularly by Penfield and his associates, because during brain surgery it is often important to determine part of the motor map, using for this purpose the conventional stimulating technique. In Fig. 4-1 along the strip of motor cortex, there are marked the general areas for toes, foot, leg, thigh, body, shoulder, arm, hand, fingers and thumb, neck, head, face, etc., starting in the midline and progressing downwards over the surface. You will note that there is a large representation for hand, fingers, and thumb, and an even larger area

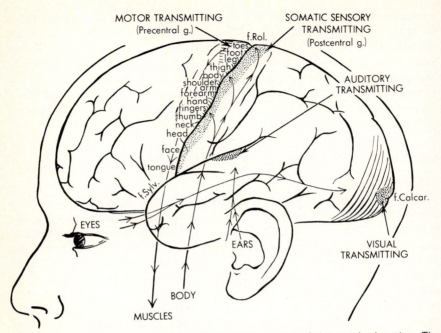

MOTOR TRANSMITTING
(Precentral g.)

SOMATIC SENSORY
TRANSMITTING
(Postcentral g.)

f.Rol.

toes
foot
leg
thigh
body
shoulder
arm
forearm
hand
fingers
thumb
neck
head
face
tongue

f.Sylv.

AUDITORY
TRANSMITTING

f.Calcar.

EYES

EARS

VISUAL
TRANSMITTING

BODY

MUSCLES

Figure 4-1 The motor and sensory transmitting areas of the cerebral cortex. The approximate map of the motor transmitting areas is shown in the precentral gyrus, while the somatic sensory receiving areas (cf. Fig. 3-13) are in a similar map in the postcentral gyrus. Other primary sensory areas shown are the visual and auditory, but they are largely in areas screened from this lateral view.

for face and tongue. So you see that the motor cortex is not uniformly spread in proportion to muscle size—far from it. The muscles controlling the thumb have a large representation, but then we use them in so many skilled actions; and even more important are the areas for movement of tongue, lip, and larynx that are used in all the subtleties of expression in talking and singing. It is skill and finesse that is reflected in the representation.

Figure 4-2 shows diagrammatically the course of the pyramidal tract from the motor cortex to the spinal cord. After descending through the brain stem and giving off many branches, the pyramidal tracts cross or decussate in the medulla and so course down the spinal cord to terminate at various levels making, with primates, strong monosynaptic connections on motoneurons. This very direct connection of the motor cortex with motoneurons is of the greatest importance in ensuring that the cerebral cortex, via the motor cortex, can very effectively and quickly bring about the desired movement. Nevertheless two fundamental problems remain. How can your willing of a muscle movement set in train neural events that

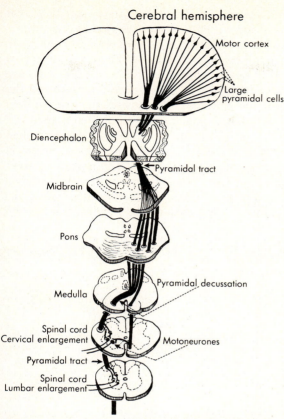

Figure 4-2 Diagrammatic representation of pyramidal tract from left motor cortex. The origin is from the large pyramidal cells, and in the medulla most of it decussates to descend in the dorsolateral column of the spinal cord of the opposite side.

lead to the discharge of pyramidal cells? How does the cerebellum contribute to the finesse and skill of movement? The first question will be considered scientifically in this chapter and philosophically in the sixth chapter, and the second in the latter part of this chapter.

Cerebral Cortex Controlling Motor Cortex

The first question has been investigated physiologically by searching for signs of neuronal activity in the cerebrum before the discharge down the pyramidal tract. In an initial investigation by Grey Walter, the subject was trained to perform a movement after a double stimulus sequence: a conditioning, then a later indicative stimulus. An *expectancy wave* was observed as a negativity over the cerebral cortex before the indicative stimulus. Essentially this wave is produced by the conditioned expectancy of the indicative stimulus and not by a voluntary command for movement. The problem is to have a movement executed by the subject entirely on his or her own volition, and yet to have accurate timing in order to average the very small potentials recorded from the surface of the skull. This has been solved by Kornhuber and his associates who use the onset of the movement to trigger a reverse computation of the potentials up to 2 s before the onset of the movement. The subject initiates these movements "at will" at irregular intervals of many seconds. In this way it was possible to average 250 records of the potentials evoked at various sites over the surface of the skull, as shown by the numbers in Fig. 4-3 and the corresponding traces. The slowly rising negative potential, called the *readiness potential*, was observed as a negative wave over a wide area of the cerebral surface, but there were small positive potentials of similar time course at the most anterior and basal regions. Usually the

Figure 4-3 Readiness potentials recorded at indicated sites from the scalp in response to voluntary movements of finger or arm. Zero time is at the onset of the movement, the preceding potentials being derived by backwards computation, with averaging of 250 responses. [*L. Deecke, P. Scheid, and H. H. Kornhuber, Exp. Brain Res., 7:158 (1969).*]

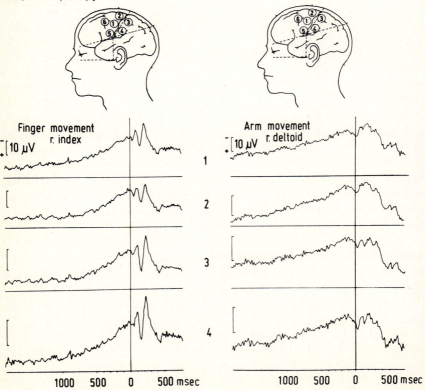

readiness potential began almost as long as 0.8 s before the onset of the movement and led on to sharper potentials, positive or negative, less than 100 ms before the movement. These were located more specifically over that area of the motor cortex concerned in the movement. We can assume that the readiness potential is generated by complex patterns of neuronal discharges that eventually project to the pyramidal cells of the motor cortex and synaptically excite them to discharge, so generating the waves just preceding the movement. The large waves after zero time are due to the action potentials of the muscles causing the movement.

These experiments at least provide a partial answer to the question: What is happening in my brain at the time I am deciding on some motor act? It can be presumed that during the readiness potential there is a developing specificity of the patterned impulse discharges in neurons so that eventually there are activated the correct pyramidal cells for bringing about the required movement. It can be regarded as the neuronal counterpart of the voluntary command. This enquiry into the cerebral happenings in voluntary movement will be continued in Chap. 6.

The Discharge of Motor Pyramidal Cells

We now wish to study in more detail how the firing of the pyramidal cells in the motor cortex is related to a movement initiated from the cortex. For this purpose it is necessary to have a microelectrode implanted in the motor cortex so that impulse discharges from individual pyramidal cells are recorded. This requirement precludes human experimentation, and I will make special reference to the experiments performed by Evarts on monkeys. In an initial operation the monkey in Fig. 4-4A has an electrode implanted in his motor cortex in the right place for recording pyramidal cells concerned in an action he has been trained to do. During an experimental run he is seated comfortably in a cage (A) and he has to move the control bar from one stop to the other, shown in detail in A, backwards and forwards in a time that must be between 0.4 and 0.7 s, else he is not rewarded by grape juice. As a variant the amount of load on the movement can be changed.

In Fig. 4-4B you can see the traces of the movement and the firing of the pyramidal cell which clearly is related to the downward movement that he is doing. Actually there are two pyramidal cells: one is very close to the electrode and hence gives large action potentials, and the other is further away and hence gives smaller responses. We can assume that the size is only a matter of proximity and not of actual cell size. The activities of the two cells are nicely correlated with the downward movement. There is no doubt that these particular pyramidal cells are concerned with a particular movement, the flexion and not the extension. But if, as in the lowest trace, the monkey is carrying out some quite different movement, like moving his shoulder, the two units are no longer correlated in their

A

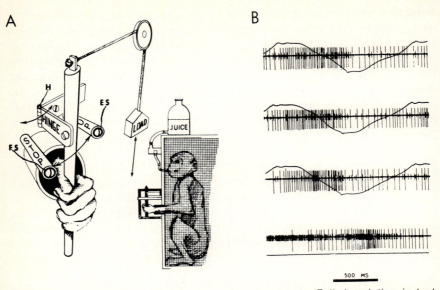

Figure 4-4 Pyramidal cell discharges during movements. Full description in text. (*From Evarts, 1967.*)

discharges but go fast and slow in quite unrelated ways. The two pyramidal cells are only correlated when they are carrying out the specific actions corresponding to their locations on the motor map. Doubtless there are many more pyramidal cells in that location also firing in effective relation to the movement.

I think this is a very important result, showing just what we would expect in the functional performance of the motor cortex when it is carrying out some specific action. There are in close proximity a group or colony of pyramidal cells whose job is to keep on firing and stopping and firing and stopping during a rhythmically repeated movement. And there would be other colonies specifically related to other movements, and so on for the whole extent of the motor cortex of Fig. 4-1. In Fig. 4-4*B* it should be noticed that the two cells are not silent during the reverse phase of the movement, but only slowed. They are, as it were, modulated in their frequency. As I have mentioned in earlier chapters, there is a general tendency for all cells to be firing all the time. Their responses are graded in frequency, coding intensity of action as frequency. Figure 4-4 is a beautiful example of this coding.

The Arrangement of Pyramidal Cells in Colonies

The arrangement of pyramidal cells in colonies having similar actions has long been postulated by Phillips because it has been recognized that the detailed cortical map defined by stimulation (Fig. 4-1) could only thus be explained. Nevertheless the geometry of these colonies was unknown. It has now been investigated by Asanuma and his associates using micro-stimulation of the monkey's motor cortex as illustrated in Fig. 4-5. The microelectrode was inserted in seven numbered tracks and various sites are noted at which one or the other thumb movement was evoked by weak electrical stimulation. The effective sites are noted and are indicated by the symbols. It will be seen that, as revealed by this stimulation, the actual cells doing one action or another, or another, tend to lie in columns

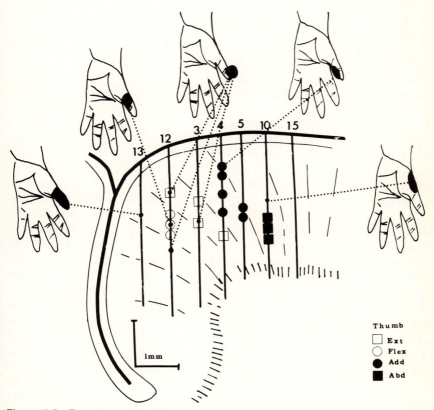

Figure 4-5 Reconstruction of electrode tracks and cell locations in a section through the right motor cortex of a monkey. Electrode penetrations are indicated by numbers and passed through efferent zones projecting to various thumb muscles. The peripheral motor effects on the thumb produced by intracortical microstimulations of 5 μA strength at various locations are indicated by symbols, as identified in lower right corner. Positions of cells encountered along the track are indicated by dots, and dotted lines join these points to the figurines of the monkey's hand on which are indicated the receptive fields as determined by adequate stimulation. [*H. Asanuma and I. Rosén, Exp. Brain Res.,* **14:**243 (1972); *I. Rosén and H. Asanuma, Exp. Brain Res.,* **14:**257 (1972).*]

whose boundaries are indicated by the curved lines orthogonal to the surface of the cortex. In Fig. 4-5 this arrangement is particularly well shown for the movements of thumb extension (open squares) and adduction (solid circles) that are produced along more than one track. There would be many hundreds of pyramidal tract cells in one such column, all presumably having the same action. It is all part of the motor map of Fig. 4-1.

The other interesting point about Fig. 4-5 is that, when stimulation is applied to the skin of the thumb at the various indicated sites in the figurines, you find out that usually this afferent input excites pyramidal cells just in the area that is the departure point for the excitation that moves the thumb to that site of skin stimulation. This means that the movement is in the sense of making closer contact with the stimulated site for the purpose of exploration. Possibly it also accounts for the grasp reflex. For example, an object placed in a baby's hand is grasped so strongly that the baby has difficulty in letting it go. I give these examples to show the simplest way in which the cerebral motor cortex could be activated, namely by afferent pathways coming via three synaptic relays (Fig. 3-13) and projecting to those pyramidal cells in the motor cortex which are the departure points for the contraction. It is a kind of self-stimulating circuit arrangement with a positive feedback control.

We can now ask the question: Why are the motor cells in columns all doing much the same thing? The reason for this is revealed when the synaptic connectives are studied in detail. Figure 4-6 shows two pyramidal cells in a column with their dendritic spines. If this section belonged to the motor area of the cerebral cortex, the axons would be going down to become pyramidal tract fibers. There would be hundreds of such pyramidal cells in any one of the columns of Fig. 4-5. What is the reason for this apparent redundancy? Let us look at the pathway drawn in Fig. 4-6 for a *specific afferent* (spec. aff.) which is an afferent fiber from the thalamus that could be conveying information from the thumb in Fig. 4-5. It branches and synaptically excites a special type of interneuron (S_1) which gives off an axon that powerfully excites the pyramidal cell dendrites by a multiple synaptic arrangement that Szentágothai has named the *cartridge type of synapse*. Thus in this column there is a kind of amplifying effect. The inputs by specific afferents are amplified by these powerful cells that make the cartridge type of synapses on the pyramidal cells. So the column gives an economy of arrangement, because the input is used to excite many pyramidal cells; hence, there is a large output—many pyramidal cells fire together. That is the way to achieve effective action. One cell firing alone is ineffective. Experimental investigation of motor cortex stimulation suggests that it may be necessary to have as many as 100 pyramidal cells firing impulses in order to evoke a movement. There has

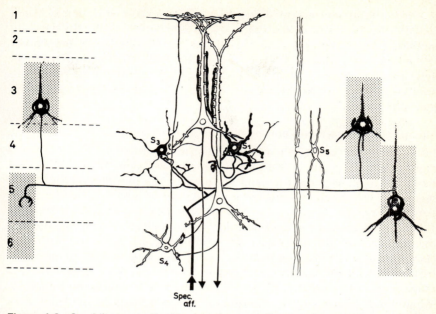

Figure 4-6 Semidiagrammatic drawing of some cell types of the cerebral cortex with interconnections as discussed in the text. Two pyramidal cells are seen centrally in lamina 3 and 5. The specific afferent fiber is seen to excite a stellate interneuron S_1 (cross-hatched) whose axon establishes cartridge-type synapses on the apical dendrites. The specific afferent fiber also excites a basket-type stellate interneuron S_3, that gives inhibition to pyramidal cells in adjacent columns, as indicated by shading. Another interneuron is shown in lamina 6 with ascending axon, and S_5 is an interneuron also probably concerned in vertical spread of excitation through the whole depth of the cortex. (*Modified from Szentágothai, 1969.*) The cover picture is reproduced from an aquarelle by Szentágothai and shows the arrangements of cells in a column, pyramidal cells being in red.

to be convergence of many pyramidal tract fibers on to the motoneurons in order to excite them to fire impulses out to the muscle.

The other operational significance of the columnar arrangement can be appreciated by reference to the other interneurons in the column (Fig. 4-6). Some are excitatory (S_4, S_5) so that all manner of excitatory circuits are activated with *self-reexciting loops*, so building up by *positive feedback* a strong excitation in the column. At the same time the inhibitory neurons (S_3) of the column have an inhibitory action on the cells of adjacent columns, three of which are indicated along with the shaded areas signifying inhibition. And so the column is self-excitatory with built-in amplifying circuits, but it also operates for its dominance by inhibiting the surrounding columns, an action that may be on columns having the opposite action on the thumb: extension as opposed to flexion, for example.

It is a general principle of operation of the nervous system that, when groups of cells are activated, they try to sharpen their effectiveness by inhibiting the other groups in the surround. But of course these other groups are doing the same. There is reciprocal inhibition with a continual fight for dominance. The result is that the movement occurring at a particular time is an integrated response and is one that is brought about by the most strongly excited pathways.

Alpha and Gamma Motoneurons and the Gamma Loop

I will now refer again to an earlier illustration, Fig. 2-1, which shows a motoneuron. In primates the pyramidal tract fibers directly excite such a motoneuron to fire impulses and so to make the muscle contract. In *B* there is a transverse section of a muscle nerve containing only motor nerve fibers, all afferent fibers having been degenerated by dorsal root ganglia excision some 3 weeks earlier. It can readily be seen that besides the large fibers that are concerned in the muscle contraction, there are also small fibers. In fact there are two quite distinct populations. I was the first to look at this picture (in 1929) in an investigation in which I was assisting Sir Charles Sherrington. We realized we had something interesting and unexpected, but we developed the wrong explanation! This was revealed in 1945 when new experimental investigations gave the correct explanation to one of Granit's pupils in Sweden. We showed that the small motor fibers did not cause any appreciable muscle contraction, but we missed the important discovery that they provide the motor innervation of the muscle fibers in the *muscle spindles* which can be seen in the diagram of Fig. 4-7 to be in parallel with the muscle fibers responsible for the contraction, the so-called *extrafusal fibers*. The small motor nerve fibers come from small motoneurons lying interspersed with the large motoneurons for the same muscle. The large motoneurons are called *alpha* (α) and the small ones *gamma* (γ) and their axons (γ fibers) exclusively innervate the muscle spindles which will be lying in parallel to the extrafusal fibers that are exclusively α innervated. This α innervation of extrafusal fibers was the theme of much of Chap. 2.

In the simplified diagram of Fig. 4-7 it can be seen that an annulo-spiral ending around a muscle fiber of the spindle discharges along a group Ia afferent fiber, as already described in Chap. 3 (Fig. 3-1*A*). The several *intrafusal fibers* bundled together in a spindle form two distinct species, and there are also *secondary endings* with smaller afferent fibers (group 2) than the large Ia afferent fibers of the annulospiral ending. Nevertheless for our present purpose the simplified diagram of Fig. 4-7 is adequate. It is the Ia fiber that gives the monosynaptic innervation of motoneurons that was the theme of much of Chap. 3.

If you pull on the tendon of the muscle, as shown by the arrow to the

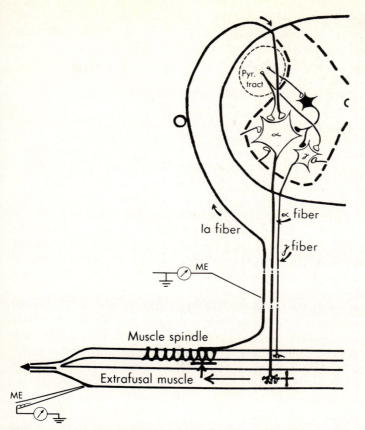

Figure 4-7 Nerve pathways to and from the spinal cord showing the essential features of alpha (α) and gamma (γ) motoneuron action and interaction. Full description in text.

left, you excite the spindle to discharge impulses up the Ia fiber (cf. Fig. 1-8A). If the intrafusal fibers are excited to contract by γ motor impulses, there is powerful excitation of the annulospiral endings (as illustrated in *c* to *b* to *a* in Fig. 1-8A), and so there is an intensification of the monosynaptic activation of the α motoneurons. If, on the other hand, α motoneuron discharge causes the extrafusal muscle fibers to contract, tension is taken off the muscle spindle that is in parallel with it and the annulospiral ending will discharge less or not at all. But, if you fire the γ motoneurons at the same time as the alpha, the muscle spindle will contract and so will not be slackened. You can see that this arrangement gives a nice *servomechanism* performance. The more the α motoneurons are firing in response in part to the Ia input, the stronger the extrafusal contraction and the less the Ia activation of the α motoneurons by the so-called γ *loop*. But the action of that loop can be biased over a wide range of levels by the discharge of γ motoneurons. There is thus an adjustable *servoloop control* of muscle contraction in accord with the biasing by γ motoneuron discharge.

The Pyramidal Tract Innervation of Alpha and Gamma Motoneurons

In Fig. 4-7 it is shown that the fast pyramidal tract fibers monosynaptically excite both α and γ motoneurons. There also would be inhibitory action via interneurons. When performing a voluntary movement, both α and γ motoneurons are caused to discharge by the pyramidal tract. The next point of the story is a very challenging theory by Merton, who proposed that the usual sequence was that γ motoneurons were first caused to discharge and the resulting spindle contraction activated a powerful Ia discharge that reflexively caused the α motoneurons to discharge with the resultant muscular contraction. That complex sequence involving loop operation has some advantages in that the servomechanism is working before the contraction starts. I will now describe a rigorous testing of this theory and its refutation.

It has now been shown in beautiful experiments by Hagbarth and Vallbo that in voluntary movement the pyramidal tract impulses excite both α and γ motoneurons (*coactivation*), the whole α-γ complex being put into action in an approximately synchronous manner. The α motoneurons are excited to discharge impulses and so bring about the muscle contraction. At about the same time the γ motoneurons discharge, so exciting the muscle spindles and setting the γ loop in operation. Because of the time involved in traversing the γ loop, the α-motoneuron discharge so generated by the Ia impulses would not occur until after the muscle had started to contract. It thus occurs at just the right time for the onset of the servomechanism control.

How did they make this discovery? They carried out a very elegant study first on themselves and then on volunteers. They moved their finger or their wrist voluntarily, and recorded both from the contracting muscle and from single nerve fibers in the nerve to that muscle (cf. the upper ME in Fig. 4-7), using for this purpose a fine wire electrode, insulated except at its tip, which was about 10 μm in diameter. They probed this wire into their muscle nerves by an accurate insertion technique. Then they fiddled around with the wire tip in the nerve. With luck and some courage, they often succeeded in having this wire electrode recording from a single Ia fiber, which could be identified by quite reliable tests.

Figure 4-8*A* shows such an experiment. In the lowest trace are records of two voluntary movements of the wrist, which are very quick, as may be seen by reference to the half-second scale. Above are shown the action potentials from the surface of the contracting muscles (EMG) and the impulses in the single Ia fiber of the nerve (Ia) to that muscle. It can be seen that the impulses in the fiber begin a little later than the muscle action potentials for both of the contractions. Vallbo has carried out this experiment several hundred times with 16 Ia fibers and assembled the results in graphical form (Fig. 4-8B). This display makes it quite clear that the Ia fibers are almost always activated later than the muscle contraction. In fact, after making allowance for the three factors below, the time differential corresponds closely to what would be expected for a

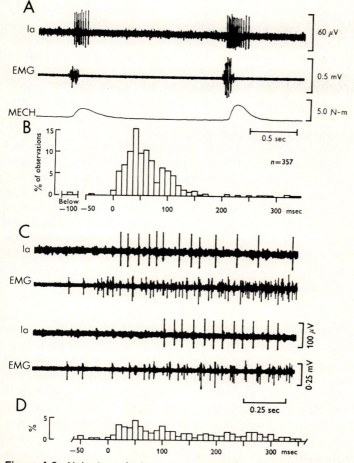

Figure 4-8 Voluntary electromyograms, mechanograms, and Ia discharges. *A* shows two wrist flexions and in *B* the histogram shows that the onset of the electromyogram precedes the Ia discharge, with zero time signaling simultaneity. *C* and *D* show slower wrist movements as described in the text. (*From Vallbo, 1971.*)

coactivation of the α and γ motoneurons by the pyramidal tract discharge, and even by the same fast pyramidal tract fibers. First, since the γ motor fibers conduct impulses more slowly that the α, the muscle spindle contraction would begin later than the extrafusal contraction. There is the additional time for, secondly, the transduction from muscle-spindle contraction to Ia impulse discharge and, thirdly, the conduction time of Ia impulses to the recording point.

Figure 4-8C illustrates the same type of recording when there is a slow prolonged movement of the wrist. In both series the Ia unit does not fire until well after the muscle action potentials have started. It is important to notice that the unit continues to fire throughout the whole duration of the contraction. In Fig. 4-8D there is assemblage of the total number of observations (many hundreds) on the 27 Ia fibers so investigated. In these slow gentle movements also it is certain that the α motoneurons almost always initiate the muscle contraction and that the γ loop servomechanism comes in at a later time, which is explicable by coactivation of α and γ motoneurons when the same allowance is made as for Fig. 4-8A and B.

These experiments have shown quite clearly that voluntary movements are not initiated by a prior activation of the γ motoneurons with *follow-up* by γ-loop activation of the α motoneurons. On the contrary, they show that there is a close *follow-up* of the γ-loop control after the initial α contraction. In considering the meaning of this physiological arrangement, it is important to recognize that in most voluntary movements the load opposing the movement can only be approximately anticipated, hence the necessity for adjustment up or down with the utmost expedition. The servomechanism operating via the γ loop is thus of importance in giving an automatic adjustment at the spinal level, though controls at a higher level are of great importance, as will be discussed below.

The Projection of Ia Fibers to the Cerebral Cortex

Recent experimental evidence has been important in revealing that, despite the inability of the group Ia afferent fibers to provide a specific sensation of muscle length or tension, they nevertheless provide essential information to the cerebral cortex on the progress of movements that it initiates. It has been customary to think that the information about the movements of the limb with respect to position and load were signaled by such receptors as those in the joints and fascia and perhaps even skin, and that the muscle receptors such as the annulospiral endings with their Ia fibers did not contribute any information to the cerebral cortex that could be used for determining limb position and movement. It has been recognized for several years by Oscarsson, Landgren, and associates that group Ia fibers do project to the cerebral cortex via several synaptic relays, but only recently has it been shown by Matthews and associates that they give important information to the cerebral cortex with respect to the movement and position of the limb. In fact their principal function may be to signal to the cerebral cortex the progress of the movement that it has just previously programmed. This is not to deny the importance of the other sensory inputs from the limb to the cortex, but merely to recognize this additional information input to the cortex.

After a penetrating analysis of these problems Granit concludes that "coactivated spindles, which are the only end organs reflecting demand and execution, play a most essential role in our judgments about muscular exertion, difficult though it be to formulate the proprioceptive experience in the way we describe things seen and heard." Furthermore Granit has shown how various illusions of muscular movements—the kinesthetic illusions—can be explained, for example, those illusions occurring in relation to postural after-contractions or the muscle contractions produced by vibratory stimulation of its tendon. The suggested explanation is that the illusion results from a perceived mismatch between the willed movement and the feedback to the cortex of group Ia afferent information. Only the unexpected is perceived with the vividness to give an illusion. On this basis Granit has been able to explain many kinesthetic illusions that are described in the classical literature.

I think that it is important to realize that much information to the cerebral cortex from receptor organs does not immediately give you some special sensation as with hearing or vision but rather something so much less vivid that it is not ordinarily recognized. For example, the vestibular receptors in the inner ear give us a feeling of the rightness of the situation. The world is as it should be. I move my head around and the world remains fixed. If this vestibular sense goes wrong, we experience vertigo in which the world is moving when our head is fixed. This demonstrates that the vestibular receptors do in fact signal to consciousness. It is the same with the Ia receptors of muscle. Quite a lot of the Ia input to the cerebrum is not appreciated normally, but when it is disordered, when there is some mismatch as in the illusions, then you know that it is getting through to consciousness.

MOTOR CONTROL BY THE CEREBELLUM

Introduction

I now come to the cerebellum, which is the principal organ concerned in the control of movement. It has been my field of scientific interest for the last 12 years. Figure 4-9A shows the cerebellum lying posteriorly and below the cerebrum in a brain viewed from the left side, and in *B* the cerebellum is seen from the top after the cerebrum has been removed. Three main components are seen in medial lateral sequence, the *vermis* (V), the *pars intermedia* (PI), and the *hemispheres* (H). It will be noticed that the cerebellum is built up from a multitude of *transverse folia*. These are shown cut across in the sagittal section of Fig. 4-9*C*, which displays how the complex folded arrangement maximizes the area of cerebellar cortex that can be packed in the limited area below the cerebral hemispheres. Note also the *fissura prima* (FP), the deep fissure that separates the anterior from the posterior lobe.

In Fig. 1-1 it can be seen that as the brain grew the cerebellum grew commensurately through all the vertebrate evolution. We have to think of it as a part of the brain designed to function as a computer in handling all the complex inputs from receptors or from other parts of the brain. It is a computer which was built, originally, in relationship to the swimming of fish, using data from receptors in their lateral line organs and their vestibular mechanisms. But in the evolutionary process it has turned out that it can be used for a wide variety of data computations, particularly in all the complex mechanisms involved in skilled movements, for example in bird flight. A simple clinical test is the familiar placing of the finger on the tip of the nose. It has long been known that the cerebellum is concerned very importantly indeed in the control of all complex and subtle movements, as in the playing of musical instruments for example. This relationship of the cerebellum to motor control was already appreciated in the last century as a result of surgical lesions in animals and clinical lesions in man. Clumsiness and all kinds of badly disordered movements resulted from such lesions. With the great development of the

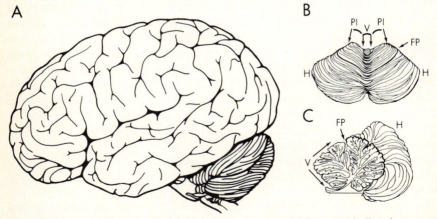

Figure 4-9 *A.* Human cerebrum and cerebellum. In *B* and *C* the cerebellum is seen on the same scale from the dorsal aspect and after a sagittal section in the midline.

cerebellum in the evolution of humans (cf. Fig. 1-1) there came all our motor skills. We are accustomed to think of these skills as being particularly exemplified by tool manufacture and usage that eventually developed into our technology and civilization. But an even more important motor skill was in being able to speak. It was this development of the cerebellum with the cerebrum, together as a linked evolutionary process, that gave the human species its immense superiority in survival.

Evidence from Cerebellar Lesions

The best studies ever made on human cerebellar lesions were done in the early 1920s by Gordon Holmes on patients from the First World War who had had the cerebellum on one side destroyed by gunshot wounds with the other side normal and so available as a control. Figure 4-10 is a beautiful example of a simple technique that he developed. He placed a little electric bulb on the finger of this subject and caused it to flash at 25 times a second. There were two columns of three red lights and the subject was instructed to point with his outstretched arm and as quickly as possible to the succession of red lights from one and the other column. Meanwhile the movement, as revealed by the flashing light, was recorded by a fixed camera. In Fig. 4-10*A* you can see that on the normal side there was a smooth and accurate movement from side to side to each red light in turn. On the contrary on the side with the cerebellar lesion, *B*, the subject gave an irregular and clumsy performance, as can be seen in tracings as he approached one after another of the target points, particularly on the two lowest where he failed badly with irregular tremor.

So, quite clearly, each side of the cerebellum is concerned in the smooth and reliable control of movement of the arm on that side. Another disability suffered by these cerebellar patients was that they could not smoothly carry out any movement involving several joints of the arm. They had to do it joint by joint. This disability is called *decomposition of movement*. One of Holmes' patients described this very well saying, "The movements of my left hand are done subconsciously, but I have to think out each movement of my right arm. I come to a dead stop in turning and have to think before I start again." This shows you how much we are spared this mental concentration by the cerebellum. What you do with ordinary movements is to give a general command—such as "place finger on nose," or "write signature," or "pick up glass"—and the whole motor performance goes automatically. For example, you don't have to spell out your name letter by letter when you're writing your signature; if you did the bank manager would not recognize it. You just give the general command from the cerebrum and let the cerebro-cerebellar circuits take over in order to give the fine characteristic details.

A

B

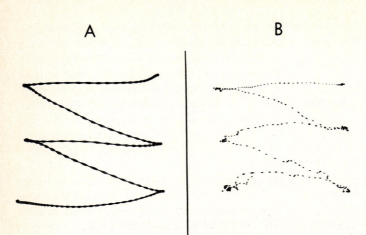

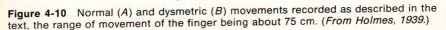

Figure 4-10 Normal (*A*) and dysmetric (*B*) movements recorded as described in the text, the range of movement of the finger being about 75 cm. (*From Holmes, 1939.*)

In summary we can say that normally our most complex muscle movements are carried out subconsciously and with consummate skill. The more subconscious you are in a golf stroke, the better it is, and the same with tennis, skiing, skating, or any other skill. In all these performances we do not have any appreciation of the complexity of muscle contractions and joint movements. All that we are voluntarily conscious of is a general directive given by what we may call our voluntary command system. All the finesse and skill seems naturally and automatically to flow from that. It is my thesis that the cerebellum is concerned in all this enormously complex organization and control of movement, and that throughout life, particularly in the earlier years, we are engaged in an incessant teaching program for the cerebellum. As a consequence, it can carry out all of these remarkable tasks that we set it to do in the whole repertoire of our skilled movements in games, in techniques, in musical performance, in speech, dance, song, and so on. Dance and song are the most fantastically demanding on your system. How is it that Margot Fonteyn, Maria Callas, and Joan Sutherland can do what they can do? This requires the exquisite finesse of motor control. It's wonderfully rewarding if you have it!

The Neuronal Structure of the Cerebellum

In attempting to understand how the cerebellum carries out this amazing action as a software computer, we are fortunate to have a precise picture of its neuronal structure, which we owe in the first place to the genius of Ramón y Cajal. It is a surprisingly uniform, stereotyped structure, that is laid out, as you might expect for a computer, with geometrical precision. It is a rectangular laminated lattice as illustrated in Fig. 4-11, where a small fragment of a folium is shown in a perspective drawing. The principal neurons are the Purkinje cells (PC), which provide the only output lines, their axons ending in the *cerebellar nuclei* (CN), i.e., these axons convey all the computational messages from the cerebellar cortex. The information that flows into the cerebellar cortex is entirely by two types of afferent fibers: the *climbing fibers* (CF) that twine around the Purkinje cell dendrites and the *mossy fibers* (MF) that branch enormously and synapse on the little *granule cells* (GrC) in the granular layer (GrL) whose axons pass up to the molecular layer (MoL) to bifurcate and form the *parallel fibers* (PF) that run along the folium for about 3 mm. Thus they are orthogonal to the espalier-like dendritic trees of the *Purkinje (PC)*, *basket (BC)*, and *stellate cells (SC)* with which they make numerous synapses, the so-called crossing-over synapses. The basket-cell axons are also transverse, traveling about 0.6 mm in either direction to form synapses on the Purkinje cell somata. Finally there are the *Golgi cells*

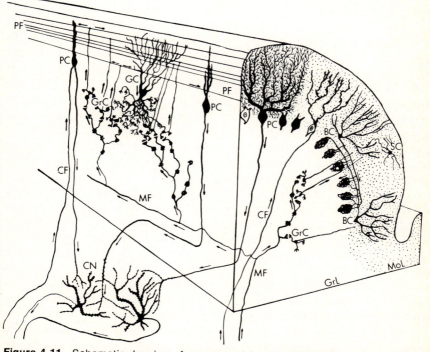

Figure 4-11 Schematic drawing of a segment of a cerebellar folium. Full description in text. (*C. A. Fox, "The Structure of the Cerebellar Cortex," in Correlative Anatomy of the Nervous System, Macmillan, New York, 1962, p. 193.*)

(GC), one being shown in Fig. 4-11, which also receives synapses from the parallel fibers and have profusely branched axons that end on the granule cell dendrites.

The neuronal numbers are quite enormous. There are, for example, about 30,000 million granule cells, 30 million Purkinje cells, and 200 million basket and stellate cells in the human cerebellum. Each Purkinje cell receives about 80,000 parallel fiber synapses on its dendritic spines, which is its mossy-fiber input. In contrast it receives only one climbing fiber, but this makes a massive series of synapses on the dendrites of the Purkinje cell.

The Neuronal Functions

There has been in recent years (1963 onwards) an intensive investigation on the modes of action of the many synaptic connections in the cerebellar cortex; the results are summarized in Fig. 4-12 in very simplified form, in order to indicate the excitatory or inhibitory function of the various elements, which are drawn merely as single units. All inhibitory neurons are shown in black. First in A the climbing fiber (CF) has been shown to make an enormously powerful excitatory synapse with the Purkinje cell (PC) that fires several times to a single climbing-fiber impulse. By contrast the mossy fiber (MF) is very diversified, each branching so as to contribute excitation (C) to about 400 granule cells, and 80,000 granule cells via their parallel fibers (PF) contribute to the excitation of each Purkinje cell. The basket cells (BC) are also excited by parallel fibers (C) and their axons go transversely to end as inhibitory synapses on the Purkinje cell somata, which are in this way encased in a basket-like structure (cf. Fig. 4-11). The Golgi cells (GoC) are excited by parallel fibers (B) and also by mossy fibers, and their inhibitory synapses on granule cells complete a simple negative feedback loop (cf. Fig. 3-11A). Figure 4-12D is an ensemble of parts A, B, and C.

We now have some basic information on which to build ideas of how the neuronal machinery of the cerebellar cortex can perform a computation. Two lines come in: one, the mossy fiber, is dispersed and powerful and it gives both excitation and inhibition; and the other, the climbing fiber, is a direct monosynaptic in-and-out excitation. Furthermore, the sole output from the cerebellar cortex is by Purkinje cells, which, as indicated in Fig. 4-12D, inhibit the intracerebellar nuclear cells (ICNC). In fact, all neurons of the cortex are inhibitory except the granule cells. Nowhere else in the brain do we know of such dominance of inhibition.

It has been suggested that this dominance is of great value in the computer-like operation of the cerebellar cortex. Since all inputs are transmuted into inhibitory action within at most two synaptic relays, there can be no prolonged chattering in chains of excitatory neurons such as

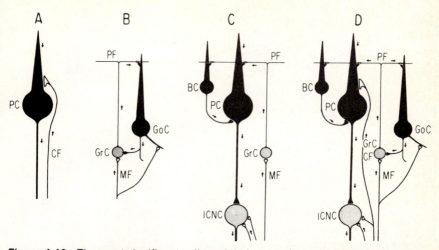

Figure 4-12   The most significant cells and their synaptic connections in the cerebellar cortex. The component circuits of *A*, *B*, and *C* are assembled together in *D*. Arrows show lines of operation. Inhibitory cells are shown in black. PC, Purkinje cell; CF, climbing fiber; GrC, granule cell; PF, parallel fiber; GoC, Golgi cell; MF, mossy fiber; BC, basket cell; ICNC, intracerebellar nuclear cell.

would occur by the Purkinje cell axon collaterals if these were excitatory. As a consequence within 0.1 s after some computation, that area of the cerebellar cortex is "clean," ready for the next computation. This automatic "cleansing" is very important in giving reliable performance during quick movements. We can regard the arrangement to have the sole output via the inhibitory Purkinje cells as being a very clever piece of evolutionary design.

So far we have discussed the excitatory and inhibitory actions in the cerebellar cortex as if they were all superimposed without any pattern, though already in Fig. 4-11 we have seen the design as a rectangular lattice. The essential pattern is idealized in Fig. 4-13*A* and *B*, where there are a transverse section of a folium (*A*) much as seen to the right of Fig. 4-11, and (*B*) the same folium seen from above as a sort of plan. It is assumed in *A* that an input of mossy-fiber impulses excites a compact group of granule cells (GrC). In *B* their axons run as parallel fibers (PF) about 2 mm along the folium exciting the Purkinje cells (PC), which are shown diagrammatically by a circle superimposed on a rectangle. Shown in black are the basket cells (BC) whose axons (BA) give Purkinje cell inhibitions on each side, as symbolized by the dark shading, just as in the cerebral cortex (Fig. 4-6). So we have here, powerfully developed, an inhibitory surround on either side of the beam of excited Purkinje cells. Thus a mossy-fiber input excites a beam of parallel fibers that gives Purkinje cell excitation on-beam and inhibition off-beam on either side.

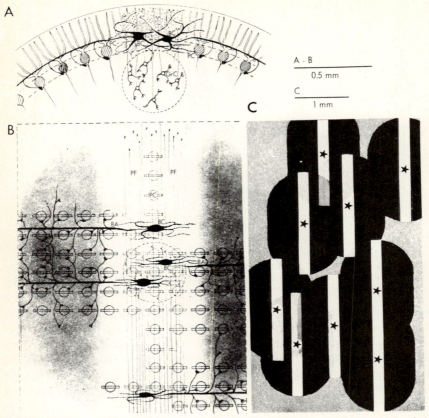

Figure 4-13 Illustration of the concept of the higher-order integrative unit of the mossy afferent-parallel fiber-neuronal chain. Neuron matrix of folium is seen in transverse section (*A*) and from the surface (*B*), with special reference to the basket cells (BC) and the inhibitory surround produced by their axons (BA). (*From Eccles, Ito, and Szentagothai, 1967.*) In *C* is illustrated the interaction on Purkinje cells of excitation by the parallel fibers and of inhibition produced by the lateral inhibition of basket cells for nine focused mossy-fiber inputs. Further description in text.

But that of course is only for a single mossy-fiber input focused, as it would be, by the negative feedback of the Golgi cells.

In normal operation of the cerebellum there would be multitudes of such mossy-fiber inputs resulting in antagonistic excitatory and inhibitory actions as illustrated diagrammatically for nine inputs (stars) in Fig. 4-13*C*, which is drawn on a less expanded scale. The overlapping excitatory strips with inhibitory surrounds result in a pattern of various levels of Purkinje cell excitation, as indicated by the shading. It gives, as it were, a glimpse of the battle of excitatory and inhibitory action on Purkinje cells that is fought all the time from moment to moment in every part of the cerebellum. That is the essence of this computational operation. No excitatory input is just allowed to have unchallenged excitatory action on the Purkinje cells. It has to fight its way through against the opposite inhibitory action. The situation is thus seen to be comparable with that illustrated in the cerebral cortex in Fig. 4-6.

CEREBRO-CEREBELLAR PATHWAYS

The Closed Loop via the Pars Intermedia of the Cerebellar Cortex

Figure 4-14 is a very greatly simplified diagram to show how the cerebrum and the cerebellum are linked together. All the neuronal pathways drawn in Fig. 4-14 are securely based on anatomical and physiological investigations. Simplification is achieved by having the individual species of cells reduced to just one example. However, each species shown has been recorded as individual cells, and the connectivities shown have all been checked by the timing of their discharges in each of the pathways. So this is a fairly complete diagram so far as it goes, but of course it misses all the operational features deriving from the enormous numbers of cells in parallel with the wealth of convergence and divergence that has been already mentioned in part. Thus Fig. 4-14 should be regarded merely as a skeleton drawing.

Let us start the operative sequences of Fig. 4-14 by the firing of a large pyramidal cell (L. PYR. C.) of the motor cortex. These cells are of course the principal cells of origin of the *pyramidal tract* (PT) (cf. Figs. 4-2, 4-5, and 4-6). There is also shown one *small pyramidal cell* (S. PYR. C.). Axons of these cells form small fibers of the pyramidal tract, but it is not known how effective these fibers are in the spinal cord. For this reason only large pyramidal fibers are shown in Fig. 4-7, sending collaterals to both α and γ motoneurons, and so being responsible for the action potentials of muscle fibers and of Ia fibers in Fig. 4-8. In Fig. 4-14 the large pyramidal tract fiber sends off branches that after synaptic relay in the nuclei pontis (PN) and the lateral reticular nucleus (LRN) give mossy-fiber (MF) inputs to the cerebellar cortex (pars intermedia). Thus impulses fired down the pyramidal tract in order to begin a movement (as we have seen in the monkey in Fig. 4-4 making to and fro movements) will at the same time go to the cerebellar cortex on the opposite side from the cerebral cortex and on the same side as the movement. So there is an extremely fast and reliable input from the cerebrum to the cerebellum. The cerebrum cannot begin instituting any action without the cerebellum

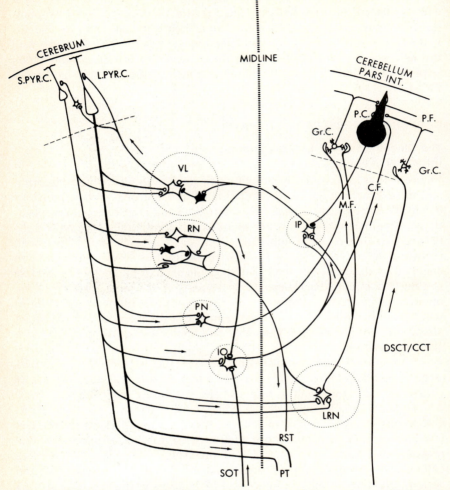

Figure 4-14 Pathways linking the sensorimotor areas of the cerebrum with the pars intermedia of the cerebellum. Full description in the text.

immediately knowing about it. There is, I think, no doubt that the cerebrum is the command center, but all instructions it fires to the motor machinery of the spinal cord are immediately fired into all the computational machinery of the cerebellar cortex via these two mossy-fiber pathways, one via the *nuclei pontis* (*PN*) the other via the *lateral reticular nucleus* (*LRN*). In addition, impulses fired from the small pyramidal cells go to these two nuclei, presumably aiding in their responses. More importantly, only small pyramidal cell discharges go to the *inferior olive* (*IO*), which is the exclusive source for the climbing-fiber (C.F.) input to the cerebellar cortex.

After the stage of interaction in the cerebellar cortex, as in Fig. 4-13*C*, for example, there is the final stage of the return circuit to the motor cortex of the cerebrum. In Fig. 4-14 the Purkinje cell inhibits the nuclear cell in the *interpositus nucleus* (*IP*), which is also excited by collaterals from mossy and climbing fibers as shown for the LRN and IO pathways respectively. Here then is a further site for computation in the clash of excitatory and inhibitory actions on the IP cells. Thence the pathway is very fast and direct, there being only one synaptic relay in the *ventrolateral thalamus* (VL) on the way to the pyramidal cells of the motor cortex. Another pathway for action is also shown in Fig. 4-14, namely from IP to RN (*the red nucleus*) and so via the *rubrospinal tract* (RST) to the motoneurons of the spinal cord.

We can thus appreciate the authority of the cerebellar influence on the course of all movements that are initiated by the motor cortex. There is a very rapid and complete signaling to the cerebellar cortex of the whole array of impulse discharges down the pyramidal tract. We can assume that the input is computed in the cerebellar cortex with utilization of its memory stores, and after a further computation in the cerebellar nuclei (IP) it is returned to the same motor area of the cerebrum, much as occurred from the periphery in Fig. 4-5. In the cat the circuit time for this complete loop would be less than one-hundredth of a second. With man it would be longer, about one-fiftieth of a second. With respect to the motor cortex this system operates in a closed-loop manner.

The Open-Loop System in the Cerebellar Hemispheres

The cerebellar hemispheres comprise almost 90 percent of the human cerebellum (cf. Fig. 4-9*B*), the principal cerebro-cerebellar circuits being shown in Fig. 4-15. In contrast to the pars intermedia, the cerebellar hemispheres receive most of their cerebral inputs from extensive areas of the cortex, such as the motor association cortex that is anterior to the motor cortex in Fig. 4-1, and less from the motor cortex via collaterals of pyramidal tract fibers (dotted lines in Fig. 4-15). This distinctive circuitry is well developed in primates and is preeminent in humans, where widespread zones of one cerebral hemisphere provide 20 million fibers passing to lower levels, as against only 500,000 pyramidal tract fibers. In Fig. 4-15 impulses discharged from the pyramidal tract cells of the association cortex pass to the contralateral cerebellar hemisphere via relays in the pontine nuclei (PN) and the inferior olive (IO). After computation in the cerebellar hemisphere the return circuit is via the VL

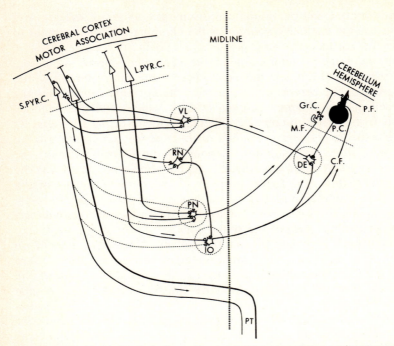

Figure 4-15   Cerebro-cerebellar pathways linking association and motor cortices with the cerebellar hemisphere. DE is nucleus dentatus. Other symbols are as in Fig. 4-14. In the red nucleus only a small cell is shown. (*Allen and Tsukahara, 1974.*)

thalamus to the motor cortex and so down the pyramidal tract (PT) to effect the movement. Thus the cerebro-cerebellar circuit is essentially an open-loop system.

Dynamic Operation of the Cerebro-Cerebellar Circuits

The circuit operations are best appreciated by the very simplified diagrams of Fig. 4-16, in which lines of communication are shown by arrows that substitute for all the synaptic connectivities of Figs. 4-14 and 4-15. Figure 4-16*A* illustrates the mode of operation of the pars intermedia that has already been considered in relation to Fig. 4-14, but it adds the input-output components of spinal centers and the evolving movement.

   When pyramidal cells of the motor cortex (area 4) are firing impulses down the pyramidal tract (PT) in order to bring about a voluntary movement (a motor command), the patterns of this discharge (the evolving movement) in all details are transmitted to the cerebellum (pars intermedia) by virtue of the collateral branches of the pyramidal tract fibers. Computation occurs in the cerebellar cortex (PI) and the resulting output is returned to the motor cortex so that there is an ongoing "comment" from the cerebellum within 10 to 20 ms of every motor command. We may regard this "comment" as being in the nature of an ongoing correction continuously provided by the cerebellum and being immediately incorporated in the modified motor commands issued by the motor cortex. Figures 4-14 and 4-16*A* also illustrate a longer feedback loop that operates through the same region of the cerebellum. When the motor command brings about a movement, this evolving movement excites a wide variety of peripheral receptors, in muscles, skin, joints, etc., and these signal back to the same regions of the cerebellar cortex (upgoing arrow) that were concerned in the more direct loop. A computation of the two sets of input forms the basis of the cerebellar response. Thus there is provided to the motor command centers an ongoing cerebellar comment synthesized from these two loops. In addition the pars intermedia has a more direct path for influencing the spinal centers via the red nucleus (RN) and the rubrospinal tract (RST), as indicated in Fig. 4-14 and by the downward arrow in Fig. 4-16*A*.

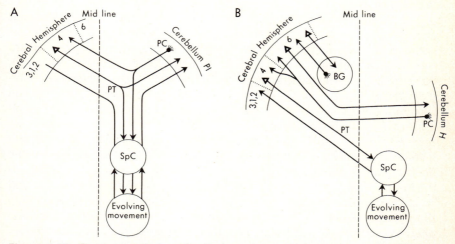

Figure 4-16 Cerebro-cerebellar circuits in motor control are shown simplified by omission of the synaptic connectivities. *A* shows the circuits from pyramidal cell in motor cortex (4) via pyramidal tract (PT) to spinal cord, and so the evolving movement, and with collateral to the pars intermedia (PI) of the cerebellum. The Purkinje cell (PC) in PI communicates (via synaptic relays) back to the motor cortex and also down the spinal cord to the spinal centers (SpC). Also shown is the projection from spinal centers to PI and to the somesthetic area (3,1,2). In *B* the circuits are shown from the cerebrum (principally area 6) to the hemisphere (H) of the cerebellum. The return circuit from the Purkinje cell, PC, is back to areas 4 and 6. From area 4, there is the projection down the spinal cord by the pyramidal tract, PT, as in *A*, and the return circuit from the evolving movement via the spinal centers to areas 3,1,2. Additionally there is shown the circuit from area 6 to the basal ganglia (BG) and the return to the cerebrum.

In summary we can regard the pars intermedia of the cerebellum as acting like the controlling system on a target-finding missile. It acts similarly in that it does not give a single message for correction of a movement that is off-target. Instead it provides sequences of correcting messages, so providing a continuously updating control by closed dynamic loops.

In the primate there is no peripheral input to the cerebellar hemispheres such as that for the pars intermedia (compare Fig. 4-16A with B). Hence, the only feedback information into this open-loop system is via the sensory pathways to the cerebral cortex from peripheral receptors in muscle, skin, joints, etc., that project to the somesthetic areas, 3, 1, 2, as already illustrated in Fig. 3-13. Because of these special features of connectivity Allen and Tsukahara have proposed that the cerebellar hemisphere is concerned in the planning of a movement rather than in its actual execution and correction by follow-up control. Its function is largely anticipatory, based upon learning and previous experience, and also upon preliminary, highly digested sensory information transmitted from some of the association cortex.

In Fig. 4-16B there is indicated another dynamic-loop system that operates via the basal ganglia (BG), which are enormous assemblages of nerve cells deep to the cerebral cortex. The principal components are shown diagrammmatically in Fig. 4-17, the nucleus caudatus (N. caud.), the putamen (Put.), the globus pallidus (Pall.). There is some projection from the motor cortex (4) to the caudate nucleus and putamen, but the principal cortico-nuclear pathways are from other cortical areas, 6 and 3,1,2 in Fig. 4-17. The further projection is to the globus pallidus and thence to the VA and VL thalamus. There are subsidiary looping circuits to the substantia nigra and to the nucleus subthalamicus. However, the main circuit is another open-loop system from the association cortex to the basal ganglia and so to the motor cortex via the thalamic nuclei. It will be suggested that this open-loop system is in parallel with the open loop through the cerebellar hemispheres. The close analogy between these two open-loop systems is of particular interest because the control of movement is disordered when either one is defective. Degenerations of the basal ganglia result in Parkinsonism or in Huntington's chorea, while cerebellar lesions give cerebellar ataxia and tremor. However, the mode of operation of the neural machinery is still poorly understood.

Synthesis of the Various Neuronal Mechanisms Concerned with the Control of Voluntary Movement

Figure 4-18 gives an imaginative illustration of the interacting loop controls. As discussed in relation to Kornhuber's experiments, the idea of a movement achieves expression in patterns of excitation in the associa-

CEREBRAL CORTEX

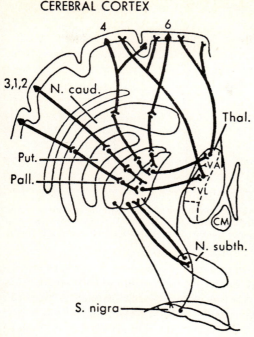

Figure 4-17 Circuits linking cerebral cortex and basal ganglia. Area 6 is the motor association cortex and areas 3, 1, 2 are the somesthetic cortex. Area 4 is the motor cortex (cf. Fig. 4-1). The basal ganglia are composed of the nucleus caudatus (N. caud.), the putamen (Put.), the globus pallidus (Pall.). VA and VL are the ventroanterior and the ventrolateral nuclei of the thalamus. The circuits to the nucleus subthalamicus (N. subth.) and the substantia nigra (S. nigra) are also shown. (*Modified from Brodal, 1969.*)

tion cortex, which are recognized as the readiness potential in diffuse scalp recordings (Fig. 4-3). At the same time there are the two systems of dynamic loops illustrated in Fig. 4-16*B* with projection back to the motor cortex via the VL thalamus. In addition these loop systems project back to association cortex (area 6 in Fig. 4-16*B*) with the opportunity of further dynamic-loop circuitry. The synthesis of all these loop inputs with the ongoing activities of the association cortex provides what we may call preprogrammed information for the motor cortex that as a consequence generates the appropriate discharges down the pyramidal tract (the motor command) for bringing about the desired movement. This story has recently been given a penetrating and vivid expression by Mountcastle.

At the stage of motor discharge, by the two closed loops illustrated in Fig. 4-16*A*, the pars intermedia makes an important contribution by updating the movement that is based upon the sensory description of the limb position and velocity upon which the intended movement is to be superimposed. This closed-loop operation is a kind of short-range planning as opposed to the long-range planning of the association cortex and the cerebellar hemispheres. Certainly both of these cerebellar zones must cooperate in the performance of every skilled movement (Allen and Tsukahara).

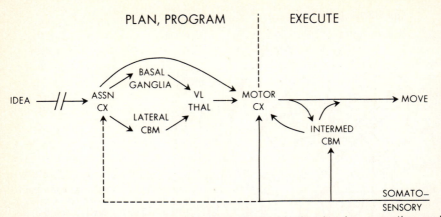

Figure 4-18 Diagram showing pathways concerned in the planning, execution, and control of voluntary movement. ASSN CX, association cortex; lateral CBM, cerebellar hemisphere; intermediate CBM, pars intermedia of cerebellum. Full description in text. (*Modified from Allen and Tsukahara, 1974.*)

In learning the movement we first execute the movement very slowly because it cannot yet be adequately preprogrammed. Instead it is performed largely by intense cerebral concentration as well as with the constant updating via the pars intermedia of the cerebellum. With practice and the consequent motor learning, a greater amount of the movement can be preprogrammed and the movement can be executed more rapidly. With very rapid movements, e.g., piano playing or typing, we rely entirely on preprogramming by the circuits to the left of Fig. 4-18 because there is no time for on-target correction by the pars intermedia once a fast movement has begun.

We may thus conjecture that trained movements are largely preprogrammed, whereas exploratory movements, which constitute an important fraction of our movement repertoire, are imperfectly preprogrammed, being provisional and subject to continuous revision. The role of the cerebellum, presumably the pars intermedia, in untrained exploratory movements is attested to by the clumsiness and slowness with which they are performed when, after cerebellectomy, the cerebrum has to function in the absence of cerebellar cooperation both in preprogramming and updating (cf. Fig. 4-10). If only the cerebellar hemisphere, with the circuits of Fig. 4-16B, is put out of action, a tremor often results because the movement is so poorly preprogrammed that the pars intermedia can only ineffectively perform its normal function, which is updating a movement that is already a good guess. Presumably the pars intermedia carries an immense store of information coded in its specific neuronal connectivities so that, in response to any pattern of pyramidal tract input, computation by the integrational machinery leads to an output to the cerebellum that appropriately corrects it pyramidal tract discharges.

Let us now try to visualize what would be happening in the cerebro-cerebellar circuits during some skilled action, for example, a golf stroke or a stroke in billiards. There will be initially a motor command with a preprogramming of the movement by circuits shown to the left of Fig. 4-18. This preprogramming mobilizes all the learned skills and leads on to the pyramidal tract discharges with the consequent report of this discharge in detail to the pars intermedia. At the next stage there will be a report back to the motor cortex of corrective information in accord with its learned skills. There will be a consequent modification of the pyramidal discharge which also reaches the pars intermedia for further revision. But meanwhile the preprogramming circuits will also be in continual action, for the movement is not just some staccato action but a smooth highly integrated performance with a duration of hundreds of milliseconds. Thus we have to envisage that, in the carrying out of a skilled movement, there is an immense integration of neuronal activities in interacting dynamic loops.

It is important to realize that no part of the cerebellar cortex knows in general what other parts are doing. All the integration of input is going on in little subsets of the cortical machinery as indicated in Fig. 4-13C. Each small zone of the cerebellar cortex is working with some subsets of the total information input, from a limb, for example, and the integration from the whole limb is accomplished in a piecemeal manner. It will be recognized that you could not integrate all the complex input coming from the movement of a limb in a single center. As would be expected, we find that the total information is broken down into subsets, so that there are many centers for many different kinds of integration. These computing centers, if we may so call them, are not sharply demarcated from each other. On the contrary they are diffusely organized with much overlap and replication in a quite irregular manner. But all this diversity of operation is integrated in the end in the smooth control of the evolving movement. It will be appreciated that it is this end result that is important, not all the confusing diversity of operation that may appear in the impulse discharges in single units at the various stages of the neuronal circuits. In summary, we can regard the cerebellum as acting like the controlling system on a target-finding missile. It acts similarly in that initially it aids in programming the movement and it does not give a single message for correction of a movement that is off-target. Instead it provides continuous sequences of corrections.

When we come to the question of the reliability of the cerebellar action in control of movement, we have to consider not only the operational character of the continuous dynamic-loop control, but most importantly the enormous numbers of cells that are involved, in contrast to the single units of Fig. 4-14. At all stages of the synaptic relays there is a convergence of many fibers onto the cell next in sequence with the sole exception of the single climbing-fiber input onto a Purkinje cell. Thus there is averaging of many individual inputs so that the unreliabilities of the units are minimized. It may be questioned if this immense redundancy is worthwhile. The answer is that if reliability can be secured by having hundreds of units in parallel instead of one, then it certainly is a biological advantage. Moreover we can assume that the multiplication of units gives in addition more subtlety and flexibility of performance in a way that we still do not fully understand. Anyway this is what has happened in the evolutionary process and the marvelous control of movements exhibited by birds and mammals shows that in cerebellar design it has paid off handsomely to go into numbers to give reliability, despite the counter-weight of all the inherent complexity. We still cannot account for the relative numbers of the cerebellar cells, particularly for the enormous numbers of the granule cells—an estimated 30,000 million in the human cerebellum. It would seem that in order to secure reliability there is this prodigious neural cost. But in reality the neural cost is low because the metabolism of single cells is so minute. The total brain consumes about 20 watts for a total of tens of thousands of millions of nerve cells. Hence, in evolutionary terms the animal could afford metabolically the prodigious neural cost, as numerically evaluated.

Experimental investigation of unitary neuronal responses at all stages of the circuits suggests that in principle they give a satisfactory explanation of the performance of motor control. But much more experimental investigation is required, particularly on the mapping of related cerebral and cerebellar areas. We have to envisage that there is some sort of topographic design of the cerebellar hemispheres and pars intermedia somewhat on the lines of the cortical motor map of Fig. 4-1. However, we know that the maps are congruent only in part. The task of the cerebellum is to blend into a harmonious whole the movements of different joints of a limb, for example, so it would be anticipated that there would be convergence from these diverse motor areas to specific integrational areas of cerebellar cortex. Tests of this conjecture have yet to be carried out on the primate cerebellum.

Figure 4-19A and B shows examples of the background "or resting" discharges of single Purkinje and nuclear cells, with the characteristic irregularity of the rhythmic responses. The dots mark the unique respons-es of the Purkinje cell evoked by climbing-fiber impulses.

Figure 4-19C to F takes us back to experiments on monkeys resembling that of Fig. 4-4 on the discharge of pyramidal tract cells during alternating movements. In D the monkey is performing the same rhythmic to-and-fro movements, which are indicated by the superimposed traces in D and F. The Purkinje cell is seen to exhibit a rhythmic discharge that is modulated in accord with the movement, which contrasts with the fairly

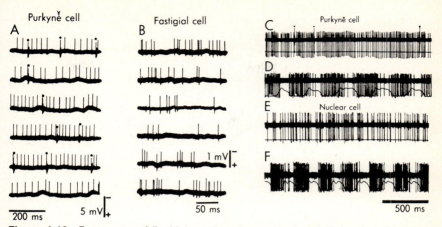

Figure 4-19 Responses of Purkinje and nuclear cells *A* and *B* showing the normal irregular firing of these cells. *C* to *F* are records from the monkey cerebellum to illustrate the firing of both Purkinje and nuclear cells in phase with movements as illustrated in Fig. 4-4*A*. Further description in text. (*From Thach, 1968.*)

steady firing at rest in *A* and *C*. This is precisely the effect that would be expected from the diagram of Fig. 4-14, and the rhythmic PT cell discharges of Fig. 4-4*B*. It shows that the Purkinje cell was related to that movement and it is explicable by the postulate that the Purkinje cell was being driven by the PT discharge. Similarly the nuclear cell in *F* showed the rhythm of the movement in contrast to the fairly steady discharge at rest in *E*. In accordance with the inhibitory action of Purkinje cells on nuclear cells (Figs. 4-12 and 4-13) it would be expected that the rhythmic discharge of the nuclear cell would be 180° out of phase with respect to the Purkinje cells projecting onto it. But we have not yet the experimental techniques to test out this simple idea. We can conclude that Fig. 4-19 in general illustrates the correctness of one aspect of the cerebro-cerebellar connections illustrated in Fig. 4-14.

Cerebello-Spinal Connectivities

These connections have been far more intensively studied than the cerebro-cerebellar connections so far considered. They are specially concerned in walking, standing, reacting, balancing and in all the postural adjustments that follow active movements—the stabilizing positions attained thereby. Essentially it can be seen from Fig. 4-20 that the same general circuits from the spinal cord act on the cerebellar cortex as those diagrammed in Figs. 4-14 and 4-16*A*. There are first the two main tracts up the spinal cord that end as mossy fibers (MF), the fast *dorsal spinocerebellar tract* (DSCT) and the slower tract (bVFRT) up to the lateral reticular nucleus (LRN). Second, there are the slow tracts to the inferior

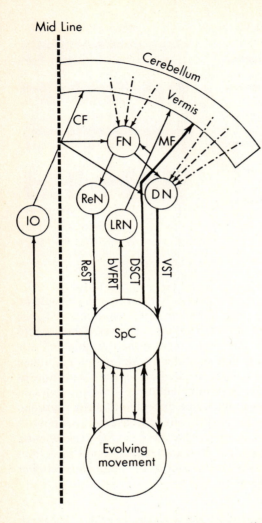

Figure 4-20 Pathways linking the cerebellar vermis with the spinal centers and so to the evolving movement. Further description in text.

olive (IO) and so to the cerebellum as climbing fibers (CF). The inhibitory outputs by the Purkinje cells go initially to the *fastigial* (*FN*) or *Deiters* (*DN*) *nucleus* and secondarily via FN either to DN or to the *reticular nucleus* (ReN) and so down the spinal cord to motoneurons via the *vestibulospinal* (VST) or *reticulospinal* (ReST) *tracts*, respectively.

The important feature of these connections of the cerebellar vermis is that there is only one loop in the dynamic control system. The evolving movement results in the discharge of various kinds of receptors that project via the various ascending pathways to the cerebellar cortex thus modifying the Purkinje cell output to the cerebellar nuclei and so via the

ReST and VST to the motoneurons. In this way the cerebellum is able to control posture and movements by the simplified version of dynamic-loop operation. We have studied intensively most of the stages in the neuronal system illustrated in Fig. 4-20 and find that the various species of neurons show the responses that would be expected for inputs from receptor organs of skin and muscle via the DSCT and bVFRT. It should be mentioned that Fig. 4-20 is a diagram for the hindlimb. For the forelimb the *cuneocerebellar tract* (CCT) substitutes for the DSCT.

In Fig. 4-12*C* and *D* the intracellular nuclear cell, ICNC, is shown with excitatory inputs that provide the background against which is pitted the inhibitory action of the Purkinje cell. In Fig. 4-20 this excitatory background to the fastigial nucleus (FN) is shown to be provided by collaterals from two pathways to the cerebellum, climbing fibers from the inferior olive (IO) and mossy fibers from the lateral reticular nucleus (LRN). It was found experimentally that the fast mossy-fiber pathway (DSCT) had almost no excitatory action on the fastigial nucleus. Figure 4-14 shows a similar state of affairs for the collateral excitation of the interpositus nucleus (IP). These arrangements have been fully substantiated by stimulating the IO and LRN nuclei and observing the monosynaptic excitation of the cerebellar nuclei, FN and IP.

Figure 4-21 is constructed in order to display the times of impulse discharges and propagations along the various pathways illustrated to the left with standard nomenclature. At the extreme left is the direct pathway via the dorsal spinocerebellar tract. Note that the nuclear areas are shown by dotted zones in the main diagram and that impulse transmission is shown by the sloped lines, with the horizontal scale giving time in milliseconds from the stimulus to a hindlimb nerve. Nerve stimulation at zero time results in a fast mossy-fiber volley via the dorsal spinocerebellar tract that reaches the cerebellar cortex in about 7 ms. It is shown with an intercept by a broken line that signifies the time delay in the long traject up the peripheral nerve and spinal cord. The slower mossy-fiber pathway via the bVFR tract is shown with a longer intercept. It finally reaches the lateral reticular nucleus in about 10 ms and evokes a discharge from there up to the cerebellum with a collateral to the fastigial nucleus. This collateral evokes from the fastigial cell a discharge after a delay of a millisecond or so, that is plotted as the downward sloping arrow. Meanwhile the fast mossy-fiber input to the cerebellum will have produced a Purkinje cell discharge back to the fastigial nucleus, as shown by the solid downward-sloping arrow. The plotted times of discharge correspond with the average values for a large number of experiments and reveal that the Purkinje cell discharge arrives at the fastigial nucleus at approximate simultaneity with the impulse resulting from the lateral reticular discharge. This is the optimal timing for effective interaction of

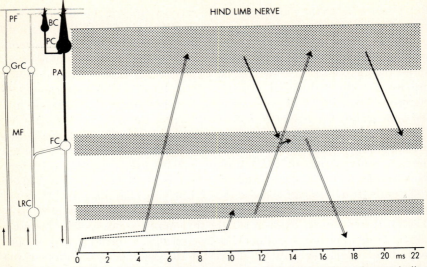

HIND LIMB NERVE

Figure 4-21 Spatiotemporal plot of impulse transmission to and from the cerebellum for responses evoked by stimulation of a hindlimb nerve. The horizontal bands symbolize the areas of neurons and synapses, from below up the lateral reticular cells LRC; the fastigial cells, FC; and the cerebellar cortex, as illustrated in the diagram to the left. Further description in text.

these two opposed synaptic actions. Figure 4-21 thus displays an excellent design of the pattern in time that is concerned in the operation of the cerebellum as a computer. It can be stated that, for the effective computational performance of the nuclear cells, it is desirable that there be approximate simultaneity of the Purkinje inhibition and the axon collateral excitation, so that there is, as it were, a clash on time of these opposed influences. If the fast DSCT path had an appreciable excitatory action on the LR cells, they would have discharged impulses many milliseconds before the Purkinje inhibition; hence, the computation would be defective.

GENERAL COMMENTS ON THE CEREBELLUM

An intensive study of about 1000 Purkinje and 1000 nuclear cells has revealed a wide variety of responses and a surprising individuality. This individuality of response results from the built-in connectivities in the pathways to these cells that are only shown in skeletal form in Figs. 4-14 and 4-20. We can assume that these connectivities are in part a result of the initial genetic coding and in part of superimposed "learned" connections that we will discuss in Chap. 5. The responses are all explicable in terms of these connectivities together with the basic integrated performance of the cerebellar cortex as illustrated in Figs. 4-12 and 4-13.

Our samplings of Purkinje cells by several microelectrode insertions into the cerebellum in any one experiment give but fragmentary glimpses of the immense number of colonies constituted by similarly behaving neurons (cf. Figs. 4-5, 4-6). However, we had earlier made a comprehensive study of the responses evoked in single Purkinje cells by afferent volleys from many nerves, both cutaneous and muscular, and had found remarkable examples of convergence. In order to preserve and develop the integration of information occurring in colonies having somewhat similar inputs, it is postulated that such colonies of Purkinje cells would tend to project onto a common target of nuclear neurons. This arrangement would give averaging of inputs from many Purkinje cells, reducing noise, as already described, and it would give opportunity for further integration of different subsets of the total input to the cerebellum. If there were randomized projection, there would be a loss of all specificity of information. It is the diversified convergence that enhances the pattern generating capability of the neuronal machinery of the cerebellar cortex. This postulate of organized projection from Purkinje cells to the nuclear cells has already been investigated by a systematic investigation of both nuclear cell responses and the neurons to which these nuclear cells project.

The relative simplicity of the neuronal design of the cerebellum together with its well-defined action in control of movement provide a most enticing challenge, both experimentally and theoretically. It is my belief that the cerebellum will be the first part of the brain to be "understood" in its total performance. For this reason I have given a rather detailed account of the linkage between structure and function in specific cerebellar performances, and of theoretical developments from these investigations. Much of this theory is speculative, going beyond what has been scientifically demonstrated. But this is the essence of scientific advance, to have theory leading and guiding experiments which essentially are tests of theoretical predictions.

Perhaps the most puzzling feature of the cerebellar design is the existence of the two quite different inputs, mossy and climbing fibers, that convey much the same information. These two inputs have been preserved from the most primitive cerebella. Yet we do not have a theory that accounts satisfactorily for this linked input. There will be a further reference to this problem in Chap. 5.

Since, as we have seen, there is good reason to believe that the cerebellum functions as a special type of computer, there have been many attempts at computer modeling of the cerebellum. Unfortunately this work has not led to any further understanding of the cerebellum. It fails, I think, because it is premature. We do not yet have sufficient "hard data" as a basis for computer modeling. There has to be much more experimental investigation using the recordings of single cells as is illustrated in Fig.

4-19. In such investigations we are, as it were, listening in to the communications of data as coded in the cell discharges, in the attempt to understand these codes. So gradually, piece by piece, we are building a coherent story of cerebellar performance. In this way there will be a gradual winning of the "hard data" for effective computer modeling. But there is still much to accomplish and all too few experiments are at an adequate level.

A remarkable and apparently unique feature of the cerebellar cortex is that its output is entirely by the inhibitory Purkinje cells (cf. Fig. 4-12). At first it might be thought that this is poor neuronal design. How can information be effectively conveyed in this negative manner? But it has to be remembered that this inhibitory action is exerted on nuclear cells that have a strong background discharge (Fig. 4-19*B* and *E*) and that most of the inputs to the cerebellum give excitatory collaterals to the nuclear cells, as indicated in Figs. 4-14, 4-15, 4-20, and 4-21. The analogy I like to give is to the sculpture of stone. You have a block of stone and achieve form by "taking away" stone by chiseling. Similarly the Purkinje cell output of the cerebellum achieves form in the nuclear cell discharges by taking away from the background discharges by inhibition. It is a challenging thought to think of this unique design for cerebellar output. As already suggested, the remarkable inhibitory bias in cerebellar design may be related to its computer function.

REFERENCES

Allen, G. I., and N. Tsukahara (1974): "Cerebrocerebellar Communication Systems," *Physiol. Rev.*, **54:**957–1006.

Brodal, A. (1969): *Neurological Anatomy*, Oxford University Press, New York.

Brooks, V. B. (1969): "Information Processing in the Motorsensory Cortex," in K. N. Leibovic (ed.), *Information Processing in the Central Nervous System*, Springer, New York, Heidelberg, and Berlin, pp. 231–243.

De Long, M. R. (1974): "Motor Functions of the Basal Ganglia: Single Unit Activity during Movement," in F. O. Schmitt and F. G. Worden (eds.), *The Neurosciences: Third Study Program*, MIT Press, Cambridge, pp. 319–325.

Eccles, J. C. (1969): "The Dynamic Loop Hypothesis of Movement Control," in K. N. Leibovic (ed.), *Information Processing in the Central Nervous System*, Springer, New York, Heidelberg, and Berlin, pp. 245–269.

Eccles, J. C. (1971): "Functional Significance of Arrangement of Neurones in Cell Assemblies," *Arch. Psychiat. Nervenkr.*, **215:**92–106.

Eccles, J. C. (1973a): "The Cerebellum as a Computer: Patterns in Space and Time," *J. Physiol.*, **228:**1–32.

Eccles, J. C. (1973b): "A Re-Evaluation of Cerebellar Function in Man," in J. E. Desmedt (ed.), *New Developments in Electromyography and Clinical Neurophysiology*, vol. 3, Karger, Basel, pp. 209–224.

Eccles, J. C., M. Ito, and J. Szentágothai (1967): *The Cerebellum as a Neuronal Machine*, Springer, Heidelberg, Berlin, Göttingen, and New York.

Evarts, E. V. (1967): "Representation of Movements and Muscles by Pyramidal Tract Neurons of the Precentral Motor Cortex," in M. D. Yahr and D. P. Purpura (eds.), *Neurophysiological Basis of Normal and Abnormal Motor Activity*, Raven Press, Hewlett, N.Y., pp. 215–253.

Evarts, E. V., and W. T. Thach (1969): "Motor Mechanisms of the CNS, Cerebro-Cerebellar Inter-Relations," *Ann. Rev. Physiol.*, **31**:451–498.

Fox, C. A., D. E. Hillman, K. A. Siegesmund, and C. R. Dutta (1966): "The Primate Cerebellar Cortex: A Golgi and Electron Microscope Study," in C. A. Fox and R. S. Snider, *Progress in Brain Research*, vol. 25, Elsevier, Amsterdam, pp. 174–225.

Granit, R. (1970): *The Basis of Motor Control*, Academic Press, London and New York.

Granit, R. (1972): "Constant Errors in the Execution and Appreciation of Movement," *Brain*, **95**:649–660.

Holmes, G. (1939): "The Cerebellum of Man," *Brain*, **62**:11–30.

Kornhuber, H. H. (1974): "Cerebral Cortex, Cerebellum and Basal Ganglia: An Introduction to their Motor Functions," in F. O. Schmitt and F. G. Worden (eds.), *The Neurosciences: Third Study Program*, MIT Press, Cambridge, pp. 267–280.

Matthews, P. B. C. (1972): *Mammalian Muscle Receptors and Their Central Actions*, Williams & Wilkins, Baltimore.

Phillips, C. G. (1973): "Cortical Localization and Sensorimotor Processes at the 'Middle Level' in Primates," *Proc. Roy. Soc. Med.*, **66**:987–1002.

Pompeiano, O. (1967): "Functional Organization of the Cerebellar Projections to the Spinal Cord," in C. A. Fox and R. S. Snider (eds.), *Progress in Brain Research*, vol. 25, Elsevier, Amsterdam, pp. 282–321.

Porter, R. (1973): "Functions of the Mammalian Cerebral Cortex in Movement," *Progr. Neurobiol.*, **1**:1–51.

Sabah, N. H. (1973): "Aspects of Cerebellar Computation," in *Proceedings of the European Meeting on Cybernetics and Systems Research, Wien*, Transcripto, London.

Szentágothai, J. (1969): "Architecture of the Cerebral Cortex," in H. H. Jasper, A. A. Ward, and A. Pope (eds.), *Basic Mechanisms of the Epilepsies*, Little, Brown, Boston, pp. 13–28.

Thach, W. T. (1968): "Discharge of Purkinje and Cerebellar Nuclear Neurons during Rapidly Alternating Arm Movements in the Monkey," *J. Neurophysiol.*, **31**:785–797.

Thach, W. T. (1972): "Cerebellar Output: Properties, Synthesis and Uses," *Brain Res.*, **40**:89–97.

Vallbo, A. B. (1971): "Muscle Spindle Response at the Onset of Isometric Voluntary Contractions in Man: Time Difference between Fusimotor and Skeletomotor Effects," *J. Physiol.*, **218**:405–431.

Wiesendanger, M. (1969): "The Pyramidal Tract. Recent Investigations on Its Morphology and Function," *Ergeb. Physiol. Biol. Chem. Exp. Pharmakol.*, **61**:72–136.

Chapter 5

The Building of the Brain (Neurogenesis): Slow Plastic Changes and Learning

INTRODUCTION

Following a detailed study of neuronal connectivity in Chaps. 3 and 4, this chapter is concerned with more slow and subtle changes in neurons and between neurons. First, I will consider the building of the brain. It is the most complexly organized structure in existence, beyond compare with even the most complex man-made objects, the computers. Yet it has been grown by a biological process in a marvelous way that I will briefly outline by way of introduction.

In the earlier stages the *primitive germinal cells* destined to build the brain undergo typical *mitotic divisions* with the making of multitudes of *clones*, one cell dividing into two and so on, as diagrammatically shown for the EC cells of Fig. 5-1A. Soon there is an enormous population of these primitive germinal cells, and this simple clonal multiplication eventually ceases. In what is called a *differentiating mitosis* a germinal cell divides to give rise to two different cells called *neuroblasts* that are shown in Fig. 5-1A differently labeled (P, N) from original germinal cells (EC). Or, alternatively, the differentiating mitosis may result in one neuroblast and one germinal cell. These primitive neuroblasts grow eventually into

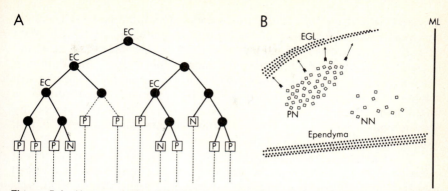

Figure 5-1 Neurogenesis of Purkinje and nuclear cells of the mouse. *A* is clonal diagram showing origin of Purkinje and nuclear neuroblasts from ependymal cells at the eleventh to thirteenth embryonic day of the mouse. *B* shows clusters of Purkinje and nuclear neuroblasts as defined by radiolabeling at the eleventh embryonic day and observed 4 days later. [*Both A and B are derived from I. L. Miale and R. L. Sidman, Exp. Neurol., 4:277 (1961).*]

nerve cells and they never divide again. They have lost their *mitotic competency*, but largely in their nuclei they carry the genetic instructions to develop into their appointed roles in the nervous system. They set about growing sprouts and these sprouts seem to know where they are going to go as if guided by an intelligence and a knowledge of the ultimate design of the brain they are helping to build. It is a wonderful self-organizing, self-developing process. This biological process in constructing a brain provides, I think, one of the most challenging scientific problems confronting us, not only now but into the future.

Two good books were published on this subject in 1970: *Developmental Neurobiology* by Jacobson and *The Formation of Nerve Connections* by Gaze. I take account of those books and of the earlier fundamental investigations by Weiss and Sperry in my presentations, but initially I am giving an account of very fine studies by Sidman, Altman, Mugnaini, Rakic, and Hamori on the building of the mammalian cerebellum.

I will now make some general statements. (1) At no stage in development are the neurons of the brain connected together as a random network. (2) Only in a few special regions has there been evidence of an excess of unused and unwanted neurons which rapidly die. Elsewhere it can be assumed that there is no redundancy. No doubt there appears to be a redundancy in the enormous populations of neurons in many parts of the brain, but we may assume that this appearance derives from our deficient understanding of the modes of operation. (3) The organization of the brain is highly specific, not merely in terms of connections between particular neurons, but also in terms of the number and location of synaptic knobs upon different parts of the same cell (cf. Fig. 1-3*B*) and the precise distribution of synaptic knobs arising from that cell. (4) The slow changes in the performance of the brain during life, in particular learned performances, are due to subtle changes in the microstructure and microfunction that we shall consider later in this chapter. In addition it has now been demonstrated that even in the adult mammalian brain there are microgrowths replacing synapses lost by lesions. (5) Apart from these microchanges, the structure of the brain is precisely determined by genetic coding and the secondary instructions deriving therefrom as well as from the medium in which the brain grows.

You can see what fantastic challenges are raised by the problems of neurogenesis. It is important to realize that the brain is constructed in all its detail before it is used. It was postulated in the 1930s that the brain was built as a more or less randomly organized structure, and then by use it was modeled to the appropriate design. This hypothesis has been proved false by the many experimental demonstrations that the nervous system is already constructed in its detailed connectivity before it is used.

We can summarize the problems of neurogenesis by returning to Fig. 5-1A. The initial process of clonal multiplication to create billions of germinal cells occurs in the neural tube that forms on the dorsal surface of the embryo. Then the neuroblasts are generated by a differentiating mitosis. With their specific genomes or genetic instructions they are already on the way to becoming nerve cells with all this know-how of growth and development somehow inherent in them. Figure 5-1B gives diagrammatic illustration of a portion of the neural tube that is concerned in building the cerebellum.

THE BUILDING OF THE CEREBELLUM

It is good to start with *neurogenesis* in a special part of the mammalian brain, the cerebellum, because, as we have seen in Chap. 4, it is a neuronal structure that is rigorously organized in a geometrical manner. Moreover it is better understood both in its neurogenesis and in its neuronal connectivity than any other part of the brain. Figures 4-11 and 4-13 give an idea of the strict geometric design. There is excellent correlation between the neuronal structure with all the synaptic connectivities and the physiological responses. We shall begin with Miale and Sidman's study on the neurogenesis of the earliest neurons to be formed, the Purkinje cells and the nuclear cells on which they ultimately come to end synaptically (cf. Fig. 4-11).

Neurogenesis from Ependyma

As indicated in Fig. 5-1A, the germinal cells (EC) in the *ependymal roof* of the fourth ventricle multiply to form a clone, then simultaneously

Purkinje and nuclear neuroblasts are generated, but the former are over 20 times more numerous than the latter. This estimate is based on the adult numbers of Purkinje and nuclear cells, and is only in part reflected in the P and N numbers of Fig. 5-1A. Figure 5-1B illustrates the beginning of the migration of the Purkinje cell neuroblasts (PN), which are moving as a cluster up towards their eventual site in the cerebellar cortex, leaving the nuclear cell neuroblasts (NN) in a cluster close to the region of their origin. Why do the Purkinje neuroblasts migrate? We could say teleologically that this migration to the developing cortex of the cerebellum is in order to be in the right place to receive the synapses from the parallel fibers (cf. Figs. 4-11 and 5-6). But that is far into the future. The migration occurs before the genesis of the neuroblasts that develop into the granule cells that grow the parallel fibers (cf. Fig. 5-2). Moreover, if radiation or viruses kill the germinal cells that would form the granular cell neuroblasts, the Purkinje neuroblasts still migrate, though to no good purpose because they are to suffer from a great dearth of synapses. These unfortunate Purkinje cells have their dendrites drooping down and are barely surviving because they have not secured their desired and needed synaptic contacts, only a few substitutes.

In Fig. 5-1B the clusters of Purkinje and nuclear neuroblasts were both radiolabeled by an injection of *tritiated thymidine* at the eleventh embryonic day of the mouse and are shown 4 days later as separated clusters with heavy labeling. This valuable technique of radiolabeling depends on the fact that before the stage of each mitotic division there is a doubling of the *deoxyribonucleic acid (DNA)* of the cell nucleus, and thymidine is one of the four constituent purines and pyrimidines used in the building of DNA. So, if ^{3}H-thymidine is injected a few hours prior to this DNA synthesis, it will be incorporated into the DNA, thus giving a radiolabel to the two daughter cells. Since a single injection is effective in labeling for only a few hours, the time of mitotic origin—the birthday—of the labeled cells is known. Furthermore, since neuroblasts do not again divide, they carry the radiolabel on their nuclei throughout life. By contrast, after a brief period of labeling of germinal cells, EC, in a clone such as Fig. 5-1A, the radiolabel is halved in each mitosis and so is rapidly diluted beyond recognition. This radiolabeling establishes that the Purkinje cells and nuclear cells are formed at exactly the same time (the eleventh to thirteenth embryonic days of the mouse), and, since they are formed at the same place, probably the origin is from the same parent cells, as indicated in Fig. 5-1A. Thus the clonal diagram of Fig. 5-1A represents the present state of our understanding. It should be mentioned that the Golgi cells of the cerebellar cortex (cf. Figs. 4-11 and 4-12) are also formed in the ependyma, but about 2 days later, and like the Purkinje cells they migrate up to the cortex.

Neurogenesis from the External Germinal Layer

In Fig. 5-1*B* there is shown growing in from the side a tongue of cells. High magnification shows that these cells are filled with mitotic figures, which indicates that they are very rapidly dividing. In the mouse the average time for one mitotic cycle is only 19 hours. This rapidly increasing zone of proliferating cells forms the *external germinal layer* (EGL) that plays a major role in the formation of the cerebellar cortex. Soon this *proliferative zone* is several cells thick, 4 to 5 being the number between 0 to 8 postnatal days in the rat (cf. Figs. 5-2 and 5-6). However, this simple proliferation of a pure germinal cell layer comes to an end a day or two after birth with the appearance of a new phenomenon. Instead of the clonal multiplication of *germinal cells*, some germinal cells undergo a differentiating mitosis with the production of neuroblasts—primitive nerve cells—as their offspring. This phenomenon gains in intensity so that after the eighth postnatal day of the rat more than half of the external germinal layer is composed of neuroblasts which form the *premigratory layer* (PM) in Figs. 5-2 and 5-6. The detailed events now ensuing are illustrated in the composite drawing in Fig. 5-2, which also displays the significance of the term "premigratory."

Figure 5-2 is assembled from several pictures that Ramón y Cajal drew from his Golgi stained preparations (cf. Fig. 1-2*B*) of the developing cerebellum. He brilliantly interpreted what was happening. Figure 5-2 is constructed as a perspective drawing to show sections along the folium (left frame) and across the folium (right frame). It represents the situation at about the tenth postnatal day of the rat. On the surface (MU) there are about five layers of proliferating germinal cells. In the left frame the small irregular dark cells (*a*) are the neuroblasts (GrN) that make granule cells. They can be identified because they stain differently and they are already sprouting little axons that rapidly grow out in both directions along the folium, as can be seen with neuroblast (*b*). These are the beginnings of the parallel fibers along the folium. They grow very rapidly and very nicely in parallel, as is well seen in the figure. What determines the direction of the growth? The cerebellar cortex has already become folded and I think that the folding exercises a mechanical constraint on growth across the folium, so favoring the longitudinal direction. Once a few of these fibers have grown, the others follow because they chemically sense each other in the way I will be describing later in this chapter. So they all grow together by surface chemical identification (*selective fasciculation*) and make by growth alignment the dense bundles of parallel fibers that are so distinctive of the molecular layer of the adult cerebellar cortex (Figs. 4-11 and 5-3). It is important to realize that these granule cell neuroblasts are genetically coded to grow sprouts in two directions from the cell body so that this becomes symmetrical with two oppositely directed primitive nerve fibers.

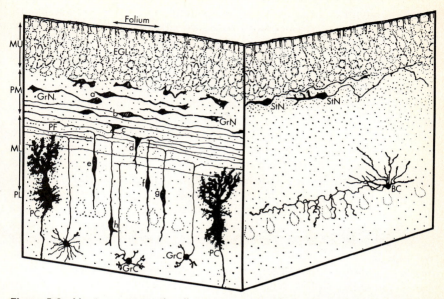

Figure 5-2 Montage perspective diagram composed from several drawings by Ramón y Cajal in order to show the various stages of neurogenesis and morphogenesis from the cerebellar cortex both along a folium (left) and across it (right). It could represent approximately postnatal day 10 for the rat. (*From Eccles, 1970.*)

The next stage is seen in neuroblasts *c, d, e, f, g*, of Fig. 5-2. When the two axonal sprouts are fully grown, it seems that the pressure rises in the soma because the protein manufacture by the nucleus remains very active. So a sprout goes downwards from the nuclear region, finding its way between the deeper parallel fibers. After a while the nucleus follows down the sprout (cf. *e, f, g* with the GrNs in Fig. 5-3), which meanwhile has grown down below the layer formed by the Purkinje cells that have already come up from their deeper origin (Fig. 5-1*B*, arrows) at the site where their siblings, the nuclear cells, remain.

Rakic has produced convincing evidence that the vertical orientation of the downward growth of granule cells is due to guidance by the fibers of the Bergman glia which are already in position. Glial cells are a major component of the central nervous system, but they are not nerve cells. They perform a multitude of ancillary functions including guidance of neuronal growth.

We can surmise that the granule cell neuroblasts descend below the Purkinje cell layer in order to meet the mossy-fiber sprouts that are growing into that location. Once below the Purkinje cell layer the granule cell neuroblast grows a lot of sprouts (i) but eventually only a few remain. The granule cells (GrC) are now fully formed. Meanwhile the mossy fibers come in and make the synapses on their dendrites. We can think that their synaptic "desire" has been consummated. It is a mutual desire. If the granule cells have been destroyed by virus or by x-rays the mossy fibers go on looking for the granule cells and grow above the Purkinje cell layer, where normally they never go (Fig. 4-11); and, apparently, finding no granule cells, they make aberrant synapses on dendrites of various cells there: Purkinje cells and basket cells. We have to postulate that all cellular elements have the instructions adequate for the normal building operation. If you fool them by distorting the situation, as, for example, by massive depletion of some elements such as the granule cells, the remaining elements do the best they can, carrying on and searching for some means of satisfying their synaptic "desire." Thus there is displayed a quite wonderful living performance in the neurogenetic story.

We now will consider the right frame of the perspective drawing of Fig. 5-2, so as to see the simultaneous happenings in the generation of cells that are oriented across the folium. At the surface there are shown the same layers of germinal cells, and below there are the neuroblasts of two stellate cells (StN) with their dendrites branching from one pole and the axon from the other. The general orientation of growth is transverse both to the length of the folium and to the parallel fibers shown in the left frame. Far down in the right frame there is a basket cell (BC) already in position. It developed much earlier, but it is essentially the same sort of cell as the stellate with a comparable genome; both are inhibitory and both grow their axons oriented transversely to the folium. You can see that its axon gives sprouts that are searching for the Purkinje cells shown faintly by dotted outlines. The stellate cell neuroblasts in the upper part of the right frame have still to mature before they will be giving synapses to the Purkinje cell dendrites that eventually will grow into the upper zone of the molecular layer (cf. Fig. 5-6).

Altman's drawing in Fig. 5-3 shows very nicely the stacking arrangement in the molecular layer that is indicated in the developmental sequences of Fig. 5-2. The earliest formed parallel fibers are below, and successive layers are stacked as they are developed. Also shown in Fig. 5-3 is the way the granule cell nuclei (GrN) descend in sprouts that search their way through the phalanx of stacked parallel fibers. This obstacle proves too much for the newly formed stellate neuroblast (StN) on the surface that grows transversely to the parallel fibers by what appears to be a series of avoidance reactions (cf. the StN's of Fig. 5-2). Evidently in their surface sensing, stellate neuroblasts display a pattern of desirability very different from that of granule cell neuroblasts.

I have described already the manner in which by radiolabeling the birthday dates of neuroblasts can be ascertained. This is best done by a single intraperitoneal injection of ^{3}H-thymidine, which gives a "flash" labeling for all those neuroblasts formed a few hours later. Neuroblasts

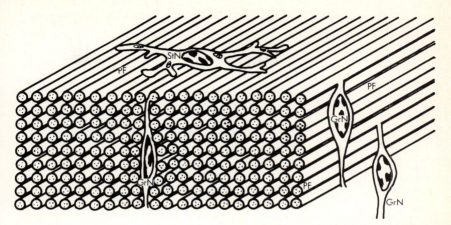

Figure 5-3 Stacking of the parallel fibers (PF) with the oldest at the bottom. Also shown are three granule cell neuroblasts (GrN) migrating down between the parallel fibers, and one stellate neuroblast (StN) growing across the PF. (*From Altman, 1972a.*)

formed earlier have no label at all and those many hours later have a diluted label because they arise from a germinal cell clone that had divided one or more times after the labeling, which consequently was diluted. In Fig. 5-4 there is a plotting of the numbers of intensely labeled cells as observed in adults after a flash-labeling at 6 hours and 2, 6, 13, 30, and 120 days postnatally. Since neuroblasts and nerve cells never divide, they would be expected to retain their radiolabel throughout life and this is shown by the very similar numbers of intensely labeled granule cells observed at 60, 120, and 180 days postnatally in Fig. 5-4*A*.

In Fig. 5-4*A* the numbers of intensely labeled granule cells are greatest for the 13-day injection, which indicates that the maximum rate of generation occurs at about this time. There is even a trace of generation at 2 days, and at 6 days it is considerable, but by 30 days it has ceased. Figure 5-4*B* shows this differential timing in the "birthdays" of basket and stellate cells. These cells are defined by their level in the molecular layer (cf. Fig. 4-11), as shown in the inset for stellate (S) and basket (B) cells. However, in their radiolabeling there is an overlapping period of 6 to 13 days. This "birthday" plot for the granule, basket, and stellate cells can be used as a basis for constructing the clonal diagram of Fig. 5-5*A*. It is in good accord with the rise and decline of the proliferative and premigratory zones in Fig. 5-6.

Figure 5-5*A* displays in clonal form the information on the neurogenesis in the external germinal layer of the rat cerebellum. The time is shown to the left in postnatal days, but the cell divisions are shown at half the normal frequency so that the diagram would not grow to unmanageable proportions. The germinal cells (GC) are identified with central stars,

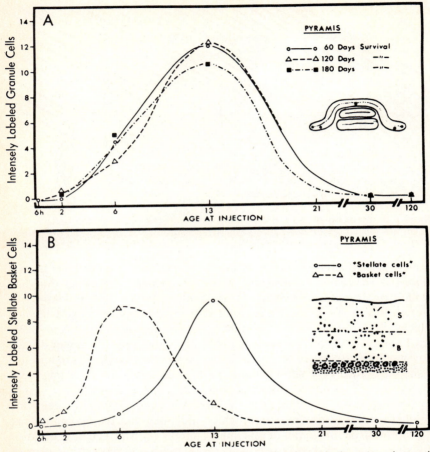

Figure 5-4   "Birthday" dating of cerebellar neurons generated in the external granular layer of rat. Mean numbers of intensely labeled neurons in pyramis region of rat cerebellar cortex in animals injected at various ages (indicated by abscissas) and examined some months later. *A.* Granule cells after the indicated days of survival; inset shows sampling sites. *B.* Presumed stellate and basket cells, as indicated in inset, after 120 days survival. [*J. Altman, J. Comp. Neurol.*, **136:**269 (1969).]

and in the earliest divisions the clone resembles that of Fig. 5-1*A.* From about 4 days onwards the basket-cell neuroblasts would be formed, one being shown by the large black circle (BN). They never again divide, but, as shown in Fig. 5-5*B,* they develop into basket cells (BC) by growing a branching dendrite at one pole and an axon at the other that grows at right angles to the developing parallel fibers (cf. Fig. 5-2). From 8 to 16 days the clonal diagram shows the granule cell neuroblasts (GrN) being made (open circles). Again these break the clonal sequence by never again

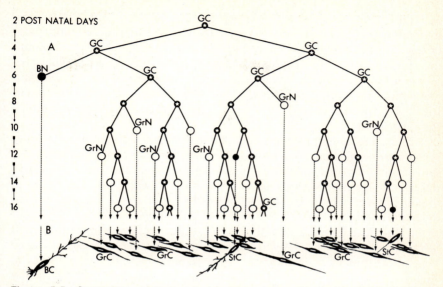

Figure 5-5 Cerebellar neurogenesis in external granular layer of rat. *A.* Clonal diagram as described in text. *B.* Perspective drawing to show development of neuroblasts to show orthogonal growth patterns as in Fig. 5-2 (see text). (*From Eccles, 1970.*)

dividing. From each pole there sprout the parallel fibers that grow along the length of the folium (Fig. 5-5*B*). Eventually these neuroblasts become granule cells by the migration down to the granular layer (cf. Fig. 5-2). Also shown in the later part of the clone of Fig. 5-5*A* are the origins of two stellate cell neuroblasts depicted as small black circles that eventually (Fig. 5-5*B*, StC) grow dendrites and axons at right angles to the parallel fibers (cf. Figs. 5-2 and 5-3). In this clonal diagram the granule cell neuroblasts are the most numerous, but this is a distorted numerical picture because according to very accurate recent counts on the cat cerebellum by Szentágothai the granule cells outnumber the total of basket and stellate cells by 80 to 1 and not about 10 to 1 as in Fig. 5-5*A*.

If it is recognized that in the time from 2 to 16 postnatal days there are 16 mitotic divisions, not the 8 shown in Fig. 5-5*A*, this figure would convey some concept of the rate of cell manufacture involved in building a rat cerebellum. It also shows how this intense mitotic activity in the external germinal layer comes to an end at about the twentieth postnatal day. The clone of germinal cells dies out because all are eventually transmuted into neuroblasts by differentiating mitoses. By 16 days in Fig. 5-5*A* only two are left. The other challenging hypothesis incorporated in Fig. 5-5*A* is that the same germinal cell clone gives rise to the neuroblasts for two quite different species of cells: one is excitatory (the granule cell) and the other is inhibitory (the basket and stellate cells). It is very interesting that in this differentiating mitosis you have this generation now of one species, now of another, with often one germinal cell to continue the clone. Furthermore I have postulated in the diagram that sometimes you can have a differentiating mitosis that results in one excitatory and one inhibitory neuroblast. This is identical with the situation illustrated in Fig. 5-1A for the genesis of the excitatory nuclear and the inhibitory Purkinje cells.

There are many problems encoded in this clonal diagram. First, what is the genetic mechanism for this differentiation of a common parent cell into excitatory and inhibitory neuroblasts? The diagram shows this differentiation as occurring as a "one-shot" process, not by a gradual evolution over several mitoses. Can this be tested experimentally? What determines the outcome of any germinal cell mitosis to be one or other of those illustrated? What sets the ratios of production of excitatory and inhibitory neuroblasts? Why are the germinal cells in Fig. 5-5A making 80 times more granule cells than the combined basket and stellate cells and in Fig. 5-1A 20 times more Purkinje cells than nuclear cells? Why basically does the whole clonal process age? Germinal cells at the onset look as if they had an everlasting life of clonal multiplication, but at about the fourth postnatal day they start differentiating into neuroblasts, and this process occurs with increasing probability so that eventually the whole neurogenesis comes to an end. All the germinal cells have been eliminated by mitotic transformation into neuroblasts which never divide again. And why don't neuroblasts ever divide again? These are all problems arising out of this early exploratory work on neurogenesis.

There are as yet no answers to these various questions, but most interesting investigations are being carried out in which some of the neurogenetic processes can be interfered with by radiation or by virus action. Mutations give all kinds of disorders and distortions of neurogenesis which lead to remarkable changes in the structure and function of the cerebellum. Fundamental problems thus arise in what we may term molecular neurobiology.

Maturation of the Cerebellar Cortex

In Fig. 5-2 the two primitive Purkinje cells can be seen to have their axon passing downwards. In fact it trails behind as the body and dendrites migrate up to the cerebellar cortex apparently in search of synaptic contacts. But the axon remains in position, ready for establishing synaptic contacts with the nuclear cells (cf. Fig. 4-11). We may call this the *axon-trailing* method of establishing synaptic contacts. The same axon-trailing process occurs with the granule cells that migrate leaving their axons, the parallel fibers, in the molecular layer (Fig. 5-2).

In Fig. 5-6 Altman summarizes the maturation of the cerebellar cortex of the rat by drawings of the situations at significant periods: 3, 7, 12, 15, and 21 days postnatally. Reference has already been made to the numbers of cell layers in the proliferative and premigratory zones during the successive stages of development. Figure 5-6 is particularly informative on the Purkinje cell development from the rudimentary form at 3 days to the almost mature form at 21 days with the profusely branching dendrites. A puzzling transitional relationship is shown by the climbing-fiber (CF) synapses on the somatic spines of the Purkinje cell at 7 days and the displacement of the climbing-fiber synapses up to the dendrites at 12 days, the somatic dendrites (cf. the two Purkinje cells in Fig. 5-2) having meanwhile disappeared with replacement of the climbing-fiber synapses by the basket-cell (B) synapses on the soma. Another interesting feature is the relatively late stage of the synapses made by parallel fibers on Purkinje cells. Granule cells formed at day 7 do not give parallel-fiber synapses to Purkinje cells at day 12, but only at day 15. Similarly 12-day and 15-day granule cells give parallel-fiber synapses at day 21.

Evidently there are many challenging problems in the Purkinje cell

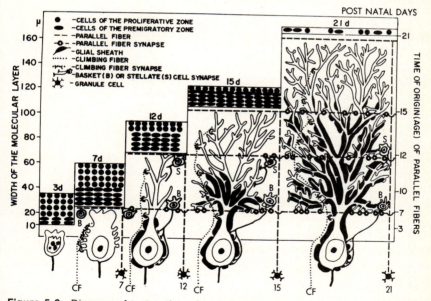

Figure 5-6 Diagram of maturation of a rat Purkinje cell and of the synaptic connections upon it. Five stages of development are shown at postnatal days 3, 7, 12, 15, and 21. The key to the various structures is given in the inset. Climbing fibers (CF), granule cells and basket cells (B) are shown at days 7 to 21. It is to be noted that four granule cells are shown with their parallel fibers stacked at successive levels according to their "birthdays," as indicated in Fig. 5-2. Further description in text. (*Slightly modified from Altman, 1972b.*)

maturation. What is the significance of the transitory somatic spines that are so striking in the drawing by Ramón y Cajal in Fig. 5-2 (left frame)? Is the displacement of the climbing-fiber synapses from somatic dendrites related to the simultaneous development of basket-cell synapses on the soma? Why are the parallel-fiber synapses on Purkinje cells so delayed in formation relative to their synapses on basket and stellate cells? What is the significance of the massive development of *glial* coverage of the soma and main dendrites? What is the cause of the great proliferation of the Purkinje cell dendrites at 15 and 21 days though no synapses are yet formed on them by parallel fibers? Apparently there is as yet no recognition between the parallel fibers and these newly grown dendrites. However, evidence will be given later (Fig. 5-19) that climbing fibers induce the branching of dendrites and the growth of the dendritic spines, and on these the parallel fibers make synapses.

PRINCIPLES OF NEURONAL RECOGNITION AND CONNECTIVITY

Introduction

So far I have concentrated on neurogenesis in the mammalian cerebellum, describing the genesis of the various cell types and the manner in which the neuroblasts develop into the fully formed neurons. Now we come to two fundamental questions. How do these various neurons get connected together? How do they know where to go? In the 1930s it was believed, as I mentioned earlier, that there was initially some kind of disorderly arrangement with usage then gradually bringing about the organization. However, on the contrary, wherever they have been investigated, the neuronal connectivities were found to be established in their final form before being used. These experimental findings indicate that somehow encoded in the developing nervous system there are enormous numbers of detailed specifications for building the final structure. This requirement led Sperry to formulate this most challenging hypothesis: that the precise building of the nervous system is due to an immense variety both in the chemical coding of neurons that are seeking to make synapses and in the complementary mechanisms for specific recognition by neuronal surfaces "ripe" for synapses. I quote from his most eloquent writings (Sperry, 1971):

> The complicated nerve fiber circuits of the brain grow, assemble and organize themselves through the use of intricate chemical codes under genetic control. Early in development the nerve cells . . . acquire individual identification tags, molecular in nature, by which they can be recognized and distinguished one from another. . . . The outgrowing fibers in the developing brain are guided by a kind of probing chemical touch system. . . . By

selective molecular preferences nerve fibers are guided correctly into their separate channels at each of the numerous forks or decision points which they encounter as they travel through what is essentially a three-dimensional multiple Y-maze of possible channel choices.

This is a comprehensive and challenging hypothesis and it has no rivals, though, of course, detailed modifications have been suggested. I think it important to appreciate the extraordinary power and the scope of this hypothesis before giving an account of some of the experimental testing to which it has been subjected. It is interesting that, so far as we know, mirror identity occurs. Symmetrical cells on the right and left sides have identical chemical coding.

Figure 5-7 illustrates Sperry's hypothesis by giving in diagrammatic form the sequences of growth of a nerve fiber that can be seen in time-lapse cinemicrography such as Pomerat so beautifully photographed in tissue cultures of nerve cells. It is easy to see that the fiber growing toward the right is sending out little searching probes. These several outgrowths at any one time are all the time probing, looking for the right kind of chemical surfaces with attractive molecular configurations. If they don't find them, they may regress or they may grow on, as in the main shaft of Fig. 5-7, perhaps getting some encouragement from the general chemical environment. So it grows on, at each stage sending out searching probes in all directions in three dimensions and then it goes on following up some attraction. In *A, B,* and *C* of Fig. 5-7 you can see "ghosts" of offshoots that finally failed after they had grown some distance. This diagram gives some kind of picture of what you can imagine happening to an incredible degree for the axon of every nerve cell finding its way to the neuronal surfaces on which it eventually forms synapses.

Sperry's hypothesis has been studied in many sites, but not in the cerebellum, which is too complex a structure for these kinds of experi-

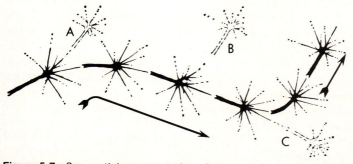

Figure 5-7   Sequential representation of sequential steps in chemotactic guidance of a growing nerve fiber. Further description in text. (*From Sperry, 1963.*)

ments. So we now leave the cerebellum and indeed the mammalian brain for the simpler brains of lower vertebrates. There is a tremendous amount of experimental work of high quality in this field. There have been many ingenious series of experimental tests beginning with Sperry's. The two recent books of Gaze and Jacobson are largely concerned with the appraisal of the chemical specification hypothesis in relation to most searching experimental tests. It certainly has been a very fruitful hypothesis. I shall now give an account of some of the key experiments in the pioneer investigations.

Chemical Sensing in the Visual Pathways of Fish, Amphibia, and Birds

These pathways have been very extensively investigated and have proved to be exceedingly valuable, and virtually irreplaceable, as preparations for rigorous experimental investigation. Initial diagrams of the connections from *retina* to brain (*optic tectum*) of amphibia are given in Fig. 5-8*A* (viewed from the left side) and Fig. 5-8*B* (viewed from ventral surface). In Fig. 5-9*A* it can be seen that the eyes of the frog look out sideways. The optic nerves from each eye cross completely in the optic chiasma (Fig. 5-9*A*) so that the right eye projects to the left side of the brain and left eye to right side. Figure 5-8*A* and *B* shows the pathway from the right eye going across the ventral surface of the brain to pass into the left optic tectum, the left eye and its pathways being removed as in Fig. 5-8*B*, so that the pathway from the right eye is fully revealed.

There had been sectioning of the right optic nerve some weeks previously to Fig. 5-8*A*. Regeneration had occurred across the nerve scar and there was full functional recovery of vision in the right eye. The significance of this recovery may be appreciated by reference to Fig. 5-8*C* where the normal spatial relations of the retinal projection for the optic tectum are shown. Thus retinal points along the solid retinal arrow project to corresponding points on the solid tectal arrow on the contralateral side, and similarly for the open retinal and tectal arrows. Corresponding points in between have corresponding projections, for example from point *x* on the retina to point *x* on the tectum, i.e., there is point-to-point connectivity.

One interpretation of this functional recovery is that the retinotectal projections were regrown in their detailed spatial connectivity. Alternatively the recovery after the nerve section could be explained by a random reconstitution of the *retinotectal projections*, the frog then learning to use these aberrant connections in order to achieve a valid picture of its surround, much as is done by human subjects observing the world for days through inverting spectacles.

Sperry eliminated this alternative by showing that the frog never learns to adapt to an eye rotation. For example, 180° rotation of both eyes

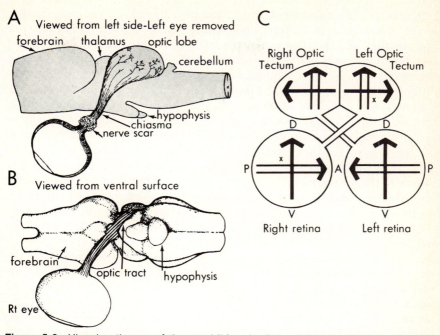

Figure 5-8 Visual pathways of the amphibian. In *A* the right eye with optic nerve is shown after section and regeneration. The left eye and optic nerve are not shown. The right optic pathway crosses at the optic chiasma to form the left optic tract that is distributed to the left optic lobe or tectum as shown in *A* and *B*. (*From Sperry, 1951b*.) In *C* are shown diagrammatically the orderly map-like projections from the right and left retinas to the left and right optic tecta. (*Constructed from observations illustrated by Jacobson, 1970*.) P, A, D, and V on the retinas signify posterior, anterior, dorsal, ventral.

without optic nerve section results in the frog striking for flies just 180° in error, as in Fig. 5-10*A*. Even for a year or more there is no adjustment. The frog would quickly die if it were not fed artificially. But immediately the eyes are rotated back to the normal position, the frog regains its old skills and suffers no disturbance from the long period of complete incoherence of movement. Therefore learning cannot contribute to the functional recovery after optic nerve section in Fig. 5-8*A*.

We can conclude with Sperry that correct connectivity was reestablished in the process of regeneration of the severed optic nerve in Fig. 5-8*A*. There appeared to be an accurate recovery of the normal retinotectal topographic relations. This finding is in excellent accord with the Sperry hypothesis. There seems no other way in which the severed fibers from the optic nerve could recover their "correct" targets in the neurons of the optic tectum. And this was found to occur no matter how scrambled was the approximation of the two cut ends of the optic nerve.

Figure 5-9 illustrates a simple experimental way of changing the retinotectal connections in a frog. Normally there is a complete crossing of the optic nerves at the optic chiasma, so that the left eye projects to the right tectum, and the right eye to the left (*A*). In *B* the chiasma is excised and the right optic nerve connected to the right optic tract so that it regenerates to the right tectum, and vice versa for the left optic nerve. After some weeks of total blindness full functional connections are reestablished, because, as already stated, there is mirror identity in the specific coding. But now, as shown in *C*, the frog is in trouble. With a fly at *X*, for example, the instructions from the visual system give its location at *X'*, the frog strikes there and misses. When at *Y* he strikes at *Y'*. The only success is for a fly in the midline. Thus the behavior pattern of the frog indicates that the retinal connections to the optic tectum have regenerated in correct pattern but to the wrong side. The frog never learns to strike correctly, even for a year of errors during which he has to be fed. So here we have evidence that the retinal specification also holds, but in a mirror-image manner for the optic tectum on the same side, giving a permanently maladaptive result. As expressed by the Sperry hypothesis, there is a symmetry in the molecular labels of the retinal ganglion cells and their optic nerve fibers. Retinotectal connections are established as quickly and as accurately as they are after a simple severance of an optic nerve (cf. Fig. 5-8*A*). There is no sign of any discrimination between the chemical specifications of the two sides. We therefore can ask: What guides the optic nerve fibers in their initial growth so that there is a complete decussation in the optic chiasma? The answer is not sure, but it is assumed to be largely by mechanical guidance and by the tendency of

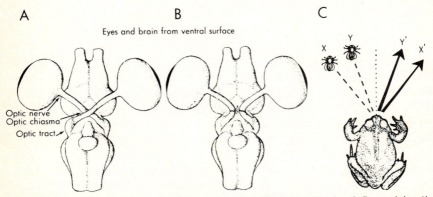

A   B   C

Eyes and brain from ventral surface

Optic nerve
Optic chiasma
Optic tract

Figure 5-9 Contralateral transfer of retinal projection on the brain. *A.* By excising the optic chiasma and cross-uniting the two sets of optic nerve stumps as diagrammed, the central projections of the two retinas are interchanged. *B.* After recovery the animals respond as if everything viewed through either eye were being seen through the opposite eye. Further description in text. (*From Sperry, 1951a.*)

fibers of like function to grow along the same pathway by what Weiss calls selective fasciculation.

More severe tests of the Sperry hypothesis are illustrated in Fig. 5-10, which displays the results of three different transplantations of both eyes. These operations take advantage of the fact that when eyes are transplanted from one side to the other, they regenerate connections to the optic tectum crossing in the usual manner by the optic chiasma. After some weeks of complete blindness the frog recovers vision, but it is disordered in the manner indicated in Fig. 5-10A to C.

Figure 5-10A represents the simplest situation. As shown in the enlarged inset of the frog head, after section of the optic nerve the right eye was rotated 180°, and similarly for the left eye. The arrows in D signify the normal eye position. When the frog regained vision, it made extreme errors in striking at flies, showing that it saw the world always in reverse and it continued indefinitely to do so. This is precisely the same

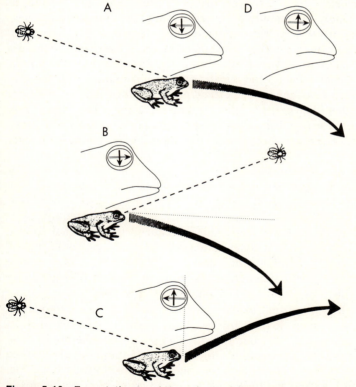

Figure 5-10 Eye rotations and transplants giving errors in striking. Full description in text. (*From Sperry, 1951a.*)

behavior as was mentioned already after rotation of the eyes 180° *without* sectioning of the optic nerves. Hence, we can assume that, after the nerve section and eye rotation, the optic nerve fibers grew into the optic tectum and reestablished their original connections to the tectal neurons regardless of the eye rotation. This result is exactly what would be predicted from the Sperry hypothesis.

Figure 5-10*B* illustrates a more complex situation because, as shown in the inset, at the tadpole stage the left eye was excised and, after the rotation as shown in the inset, it was substituted for the right eye and its optic nerve was sutured to the right optic nerve, and vice versa for the right eye. Again vision was regained after several weeks, but the adult frog now suffered from a visual world seen upside down, the vertical axis being reversed (see inset). It only could successfully strike at flies in the horizontal plane (the dotted line). Those above were struck at below, as in the illustration. The inset shows the actual position of the eye axes, and this systematic error again is in accord with prediction that the retinal maps are accurately reconstituted in their tectal projection, regardless of the fact that the eyes have been transposed.

Figure 5-10*C* shows another experiment of eye transplantation. Now after recovery the frog suffers from an anterior-posterior inversion of its visual field as indicated in the illustration and its inset. It now only succeeds in correct striking in the vertical plane (dotted line). Again this is precisely what would be expected for a reconstruction of the retinal-tectal connections in accord with the original spatial relations. In all these cases the unfortunate frogs never learn to correct their errors and are kept alive by artificial feeding.

These behavioral experiments have been confirmed by many investigators and have been carried out on several species of amphibia and fish with essentially the same results. Many finer variants have also been tried by Sperry such as excision of small patches of the optic tectum after regeneration had been established. These localized lesions resulted in a localized blind spot in the corresponding part of the visual field just as occurs normally. Evidently after regeneration there was an orderly map-like projection of the regenerated fibers to the tectum reestablishing the normal point-to-point projection indicated in Fig. 5-8*C*.

However, it is important to use more rigorous testing techniques in order to establish finer details. In the goldfish Sperry excised various segments of the retina, then cut the optic nerve. It regenerated in the medial zone of the tectum when the dorsal part of the retina was removed (Fig. 5-11*A*) and in the lateral zone after ablation of the ventral retina (Fig. 5-11*B*). So histologically the fibers can be seen finding the right places in the optic tectum. Again in Fig. 5-11*C* the posterior part of the retina regenerated selectively into the anterior part of the tectum. Of particular

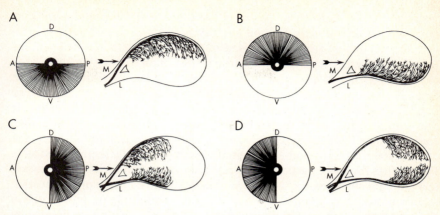

Figure 5-11 Regeneration patterns of retinal halves to optic tract and optic tectum. As in Fig. 5-8, P, A, D, and V signify posterior, anterior, dorsal, and ventral on the retina. M and L signify medial and lateral aspects of the tectum. Further description in text. [*D. Attardi and R. W. Sperry, Exp. Neurol., 7:46 (1963).*]

interest was the regeneration after excision of the posterior part of the retina. The retina correctly regenerated into the posterior tectum (Fig. 5-11*D*) and on the way grew past all of the cells of the anterior tectum despite their demand for synapses due to the fact that they, like all the tectal cells, had been denuded. Nevertheless the anterior retinal fibers bypassed them and made endings just in the right place. We must conclude that those fibers growing out from the retina are guided by a specific sensing mechanism giving precise information on the correct neuronal surfaces on which to establish synaptic contacts. The outgrowing fibers grow in a stream over the tectal surface plunging down when in the correct zone, as indicated in Fig. 5-11*D*. Cowan has performed similar experiments on the regeneration of the chick retinotectal connections. Radio-tracer investigations showed them to be reestablished to the correct tectal sites exactly in accord with the Sperry hypothesis.

Gaze and Jacobson have used electrophysiological field analysis to map the relationship between retina and tectum. Microelectrode recording has been carried out from a grid of tectal sites and for each the corresponding retinal point has been determined by scanning the retina with a light spot. The retinotectal relationships shown in Fig. 5-8*C* were mapped in this way. This technique has been used to test the retinotectal projections that were reestablished after various operative procedures as in Figs. 5-9 and 5-10. In general there has been good confirmation of the regenerative pattern given by the original behavioral experiments. There were minor discrepancies. On the whole, the longer the time allowed for regeneration, the more the "correct" pattern was established. Detailed study of several regenerating processes has shown that there is a reshuffling of synapses, the "correct" synapses replacing the less "correct" ones that had been formed initially.

Further investigation has raised interesting questions. Jacobson has found that if you rotate the eyes through 180° at an early embryonic stage of the amphibian *Xenopus*, before any retinotectal connections have been formed, the retinal fibers grow to the correct places on the optic tectum so that the toad develops normal vision despite the rotation. For this to occur the rotation has to be performed before a critical embryonic age. Jacobson has defined the critical period within 10 hours (h). If later, the 180° rotation is expressed in the retinal outgrowth to the tectum, just as in Fig. 5-10A. It was of particular interest to discover that this critical period spanned the time of the differentiating mitosis of the neuroblasts that develop into retinal ganglion cells. When there are only germinal cells in the embryonic retina, any rotation it may undergo is without influence on the specification of retinal neuroblasts formed at subsequent mitoses. But, at the time of the differentiating mitosis that results in the generation of retinal ganglion cells, the situation is transformed. The ganglion cell neuroblasts then receive their chemical coding giving them the precise instructions for the tectal location to which they must grow. This of course occurs before the onset of the actual fiber outgrowths from the retinal ganglion cells to the tectum. It is certainly a remarkable discovery that the complete coding of the retinal neuroblasts is established in the 10 h during the last neurogenesis and that this coding is somehow given by the orientation of the eye in the head at that time.

It must be pointed out that we have no idea how the position of the eye in the head can result in the specification of the retinal ganglion cells. Again there is no answer to the question: How does it come about that there is a complementary specification of the tectal neurons, matching that of the fibers growing out from the retina? Yoon has demonstrated that this complementary specification remains unchanged when rectangular slabs of the goldfish tectum are excised, rotated or inverted and then reinnervated. Again, as already mentioned, mechanical guidance must play an important part in the massive control needed for ensuring a complete decussation in the optic chiasma and in fact in the general establishment of the whole pathway from retina to tectum. Chemical specification need only operate at the last stage of the growth in insuring that the "correct" synaptic connections are established.

Neuronal Connectivity in Mammals

I have chosen to deal at length with the visual pathways of amphibia and fish because they are the best exemplars of investigations on the factors determining the establishment of neuronal connections in the brain. There has been an immense range of such investigations using techniques such as limb transplantation, skin transplantation, and cross-union of various nerves to limb muscles by a technique similar to that of Fig. 5-9. Many of these experiments have been carried out on mammals. There is always the hope that operative procedures may help disabled patients by utilizing one or more nerves to reinnervate muscles deprived of their normal innervation. There is almost no specification in the innervation of muscles. Any set of motoneurons via their motor axons (cf. Fig. 3-1) will establish functional endplates on denervated muscle fibers and excite them effectively. However, in mammals this innervation of some extraneous muscle does not result in any change in the central connections onto these motoneurons. We performed nerve cross-union on kittens a few days after birth, but even after many months we found very few significant changes in the monosynaptic connections onto motoneurons (cf. Fig. 3-1) that thus were given an inverted function.

It is important to realize that after an early stage in the mammalian brain there is no regeneration of severed pathways. There is no trace of the incredible reconstitution of pathways observed in the amphibian or fish retinotectal pathways. Yet it can be presumed that, in the embryonic mammal, the growth of nerve fibers and the establishment of precise topographical maps such as that of motor cortex to muscle (Fig. 4-1) was effected by chemical specification of the outgrowing fibers of the pyramidal tract. The tragedy for the paraplegic patient is that all this embryonic know-how is lost and the severed fibers of his pyramidal tract (cf. Fig. 4-2) cannot regenerate along spinal cord pathways that were precisely traversed in the embryo. Such regeneration of the spinal cord is possible in the fully grown fish and many amphibia. Can this embryonic know-how be recovered in the adult mammal and even in man? An encouraging answer to this question may eventuate from intensive and comprehensive investigations into the many factors that initially entered into the building of the nervous system. Undoubtedly the Sperry hypothesis of chemical specification is the principal factor, but many other factors play an important role, such as mechanical guidance, selective fasciculation, temporal sequences, and competition for synaptic sites.

The elegant experiments of Wiesel and Hubel on kittens illustrate the complexities of the factors concerned in establishing and maintaining neuronal connectivities in the mammalian brain. It is some days after birth before kittens open their eyes; nevertheless at birth the retina is connected with detailed topography to the visual cortex in the adult pattern, much as with the amphibian retinotectal connectivity. Moreover the orientational sensitivity of neurons in their columnar arrangements can be demonstrated as in Fig. 6-5 for the adult. Here we have an excellent illustration of the establishment of precise patterned connections from eye to brain prior to usage. We may assume that this is due in large part to the operation of chemical specification similar to that for amphibia and fish. But, if this beautifully grown structure is not used for some weeks after the time the kitten normally opens its eyes, it becomes disorganized, the destruction being permanent. Use by patterned vision is essential for stabilizing this fragile organization of retinocortical connectivities that presumably is grown largely by chemical specification as in fish and amphibia.

In the last few years many remarkable investigations have established beyond all doubt that a very effective regeneration occurs in the mammalian brain, even in the adult. However, these regenerations differ from the regenerations of pathways in lower vertebrates in that the regeneration occurs only for very short distances—perhaps for no more than 50 μm. Such regenerations have been demonstrated in many regions of the mammalian brain: the septal nuclei, the hippocampus, the red nucleus, the lateral geniculate nucleus, the superior colliculus, the visual cortex.

This work on the higher levels of the brain can best be illustrated by the fine work of Raisman and associates on neurons of the septal nuclei in the diencephalon, which provide ideal experimental conditions (Fig. 5-12). The two principal inputs to these nuclei are the fimbrial pathway from the hippocampus and the medial forebrain bundle (MFB) from the hypothalamus. The former input synapses almost exclusively on the dendrites of septal cells, while the latter input ends on both dendrites and somata (Fig. 5-12A).

After sectioning of either pathway in adult rats there was within a few days the usual degeneration and disappearance of the synapses formed by that pathway. Electron microscopic observations revealed that the number of synapses was reduced almost to half, but some 30 days later the full population was restored. It was shown that this restoration was due to sprouting of the fibers of the other pathway, the sprouts growing to form new synapses that occupied the vacated synaptic sites, as illustrated in Fig. 5-12B and C. In the electron micrographs it could be seen that, some weeks after sectioning of the MFB, the fimbrial fibers occupied a considerable number of synapses on the somata of the septal neurons, as is illustrated in Fig. 5-12C. Conversely, after section of the fimbrial pathway, there was evidence that the fibers of the MFB sprouted to form many new synapses, which often had the double configuration shown in Fig. 5-12B. These new synapses were all on the dendrites, which is the site of the vacated fimbrial synapses.

It appears that there has been a loss of the embryonic growth specificity, so that collaterals growing from the intact axons now *heterotypically* innervate synaptic sites originally reserved for and occupied by the other input. It may therefore result in functional disorder, but our

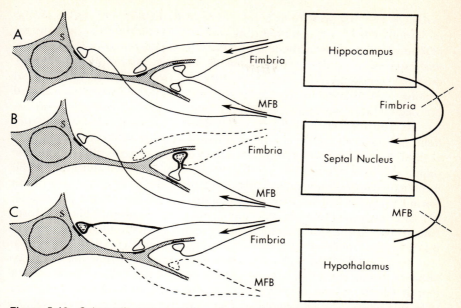

Figure 5-12   Schematic representation of synaptic connections to septal cells. *A*. In the normal situation, afferents from the medial forebrain bundle (MFB) terminate in boutons on the cell soma (S) and on dendrites, and the fimbrial fibers (fimb) are restricted in termination to the dendrites. *B*. Several weeks after a lesion of the fimbria, the medial forebrain bundle fiber terminals extend across from their own sites to occupy the vacated sites, thus forming double synapses. (Degenerated connections are shown with discontinuous lines, presumed plastic changes with heavy black line.) *C*. Several weeks after a lesion of the medial forebrain bundle, the fimbrial fibers now give rise to terminals occupying somatic sites, which are presumably those vacated as a result of the former lesion. [*Modified from G. Raisman, Br. Res., **14:25** (1969)*.]

present interest is the demonstration that axonal sprouting and synaptic regeneration can occur in the adult rat, though probably only for minute distances of 50 μm or so. In the various stages of the synaptic degeneration astroglia ingest the degenerating synaptic knobs and temporarily occupy the vacated synaptic site until ejected by the new ingrowing sprouts with their synaptic knobs. We may ask two questions: How is the sprouting initiated? How is the sprout guided to the vacated synaptic site? Rakic's demonstration of the role of glia in neuronal development makes it probable that astroglia are responsible for the regenerative growths illustrated in Fig. 5-12*B* and *C*. The astroglia are metabolically involved in the degenerating process with their ingestion of the synaptic knobs, so it is conjectured that they are able to provide chemical instructions that trigger the growth of sprouts and guide them to the vacated synaptic sites.

It has been shown in several investigations that the regenerated synapses are functionally effective, generating EPSPs and the discharge of impulses by the reinnervated neurons. Nevertheless this heterotypic regeneration may not provide a functional compensation for the lesion— and even may be deleterious. However, this regeneration of synapses must be considered in a context different from the massive surgical lesions such as those of Fig. 5-12, where all synaptic inputs of one kind are degenerated, so eliminating opportunity for *homotypic regeneration*. Let us consider instead the few scattered degenerations arising from neuronal death during aging or from minor cerebral lesions. Under such conditions we can conjecture that homotypic regeneration would be dominant, as indicated in Fig. 5-13. Thus the disability suffered by the brain as a result of neuronal death would arise merely from the loss of the normal convergence number, by which one means the number of neurons of any one species converging synaptically upon a neuron. This loss (from four to two in Fig. 5-13) would result in some coarsening of the grain in the control of neurons, but would not impair their overall effectiveness.

The investigations in many sites in the mammalian brain certainly show that under appropriate conditions there is an effective new growth compensating for the death of neurons and their synapses. It is therefore with optimism that one reassesses the often enigmatic and ambiguous clinical findings described during stages of recovery from lesions of the human brain. The most remarkable account of this has recently been given by Brodal, a distinguished neuroanatomist, who suffered a vascular accident in his right cerebral cortex and made a quite remarkable recovery in a year or two, as has been fully described in a paper he has published. Apart from such sudden lesions, we are continually suffering from random neuronal death and we have no way of replacing our neuronal population. However, this new story of synaptic regeneration shows that the brain can go on functioning reasonably well with the disability of a less fine grain despite losses which may even halve the neuronal population, which does occur in the frontal cortex by 90 years of age.

Chemical Specification of Neurons

In the first chapter I briefly discussed the chemical structure of the surface membrane of nerve fibers, and it was illustrated diagrammatically in Fig. 1-12. The features of present interest are the specific proteins or other macromolecules there shown attached to the outer surface of the membrane or partly penetrating the bimolecular leaflet of phospholipids. We can imagine that these macromolecules are responsible for the chemical labeling of the neurons. We can assume that the specificity resides in the surfaces that these macromolecules present to other neurons in the environment of that neuron or nerve fiber. This property

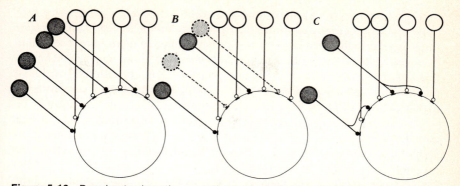

Figure 5-13 Drawing to show the synaptic terminals that are made on a neuron by two sets of afferent pathways. In *B* there is degeneration of half of the fibers of one set. In *C*, there is occupation of the vacated synaptic sites by the remaining fibers of that set (homotypic regeneration) rather than by the fibers of the other set (heterotypic regeneration).

could reside with the macromolecules as individuals, or alternatively with the patterned arrangement of the macromolecules as well. It will be an immense task for microneurochemistry to identify these macromolecules and to discover how they give to the surface of the neuron the chemical specifications which, as we have seen, play such a vital role in the building of the brain.

Moreover there are the additional tasks of discovering how these specific proteins and other macromolecules are manufactured by the neurons and how they come to be on the surface of nerve fibers far removed from the neuronal soma, which is the presumed site of their manufacture. It will be our general postulate that in the differentiating neurogenesis the neuroblast receives a genetic coding that gives it the potentiality to manufacture these specific tagging macromolecules. These are most complex problems in molecular neurobiology and can only be defined in quite general terms at present. However it is known that genetic defects result in failures of neuronal organization such as has been described by Sidman in the "reeler" mice and by Brenner in *Ascaris*. A secondary problem concerns the manner in which macromolecules manufactured by the neuron are distributed from the presumed site of manufacture in the neuronal soma. It is the problem generally known as *axon transport*.

Chemical Transport along Nerve Fibers: Axoplasmic Flow

The earlier experiments of Weiss demonstrated flow along nerve fibers by observing the damming up of material proximal to a ligature. In that way it was possible to derive approximate measures for flow of material along axons and to derive a rate of about 1 mm/day, which was supported by radio-tracer labeling experiments. However, much faster transportation rates have now been measured by improvements in technique, particularly in giving localized radio-tracer injections close to the nerve cells and by keeping the nerve fibers under good physiological conditions. I will base my account largely on the most attractive story that emerges from the investigations of Ochs on mammalian nerve.

Ochs injects *tritiated leucine* or *tritiated lysine* into a dorsal root ganglion of the spinal cord (arrow at G in Fig. 5-14*B*), and shows that the ganglion cells pick up the amino acid and build it into proteins and polypeptides. These tritiated macromolecules can be followed by radio-tracer techniques and shown to move along the nerve fibers in both directions from the ganglion, out to the periphery and centrally up the spinal cord. In Fig. 5-14*A* there are plotted a series of experiments in

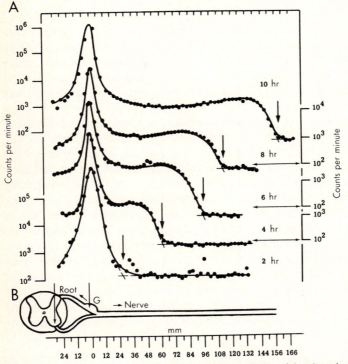

Figure 5-14 Fast axon transport down sensory fibers. A lumbar dorsal root ganglion, G, of the cat was injected with tritiated leucine and the radioactivity was measured in separate experiments at 2, 4, 6, 8, and 10 h later at the distances shown along the sciatic nerve. The radioactivity is plotted on a logarithmic scale in counts per minute (CPM), with separate scales as shown for each of the curves. Further description in text. (*From Ochs, 1972b.*)

which there was termination at the indicated hours. Counts per minute were measured for the successive 2-mm lengths into which the nerve was cut and are plotted on the logarithmic scale. The arrows indicate the sites of the wave fronts at the post-injection times of 2, 4, 6, 8, and 10 h. In this way the wave front of increased radioactivity was observed to travel along the nerve at the surprisingly fast velocity of 400 mm/day, and this speed is the same for mammals with a size range from rat to goat. It seems to be a basic biological speed in these axons and of quite extraordinary efficiency. So proteins and other macromolecules manufactured in the perinuclear region of the soma are transported down along the axon. We can assume that this transport is concerned with establishing and maintaining the chemical coding all the way along the nerve fiber. The transport is not down the spaces between the nerve fibers because the labeled macromolecules are shown by autoradiography to be inside the nerve fibers.

The remarkable feature of Fig. 5-14 is that the wave front moves bodily forwards hour by hour. If it were due to some diffusional process, the wave front would become progressively more spread out. Evidently there is some highly organized transport mechanism. It has long been known that nerve fibers are not just tubes filled with some protein jelly, but that they contain many fine structures, *neurofibrils* and *neurotubules* that run along their length (cf. Fig. 1-19*A*). It is postulated by Ochs that after manufacture in the cell body the macromolecules are loaded onto these tubules and fibrils and travel along by some sliding mechanism, hence the uniform rate. Thus the rapid transport of 400 mm/day is envisaged as being due to a "conveyor-belt" operation.

It is interesting that this transport goes at about the same velocity central from the ganglion cells and up the tract fibers (cf. Figs. 1-6, 3-13). There is a similar transport in motor nerve fibers. We can predict that it will be found to occur in all nerve fibers both peripheral and central.

An important discovery was that this transport was dependent upon metabolism of the nerve. It was not due to some pressure exerted from the nerve cell, but, as would be expected from the sliding filament hypothesis, each segment of the nerve had to provide the energy for the transport. Figure 5-15*A* shows that local anoxia of the segment results in a failure of transport and a banking-up proximal to the block. Again the same enzyme poisons—cyanide, azide, and dinitrophenol—block the transport along the fiber and the ionic pumping across its membrane. In Fig. 5-15*B* poisoning by cyanide along the whole length of the nerve fiber at 3 h after the injection completely blocked the transport. The distribution of radioactivity remained frozen at the 3-h position (cf. Fig. 5-14*A*). A thorough experimental study of this fast transport shows that in every respect the observations are in accord with the hypothesis that the

fast transport is due to active transport machinery that is dependent on energy provided by *adenosine triphosphate* and that it is distributed along the whole length of nerve fibers.

The muscles of a limb can be classified in general as fast and slow contracting, the former being for quick movements, the later for maintenance of posture. Several years ago we showed that when the nerves to these muscles were severed and cross-united, the contractions of the muscles also crossed over, the fast becoming slow and the slow fast. It was postulated that this was caused by specific substances manufactured in the motoneurons that traveled down the axons and so across the neuromuscular synapse (Fig. 2-1*A*) to the muscle fiber. An alternative and perhaps supplementary hypothesis is that the speed of muscle contraction is modified by the frequency of discharge of impulses from the motoneurons. The hypothesis that motoneurons control the speed of muscle contractions can now be much more precisely defined because it has been shown first by Buller and Mommaerts and later by Barany and Close that the cross innervation results in changes in the contractile protein, *myosin*, of the reinnervated muscles. The changed speed of the muscle contraction results from the change in the kinetic properties of the *adenosine triphosphatase* of the myosin. This finding is perhaps the best documented example of the transsynaptic production of changes in physiological and biochemical properties. It is an attractive hypothesis that these changes are produced by the transport of specific macromolecules down the motor axons and then across the neuromuscular synapses to the muscle fibers. It would be a remarkable discovery to identify these specific macromolecules.

Besides the subtle changes in the myosin and the associated changes in the speed of muscular contraction, innervation has more profound influences on muscle. These are displayed when muscle is deprived of innervation. In a day or so it changes its properties, the sensitivity to ACh spreading over the whole surface from the extremely localized site characteristic of normal muscle (Fig. 2-4). Moreover spasmodic twitches occur in the individual muscle fibers and the muscle wastes progressively, eventually to become replaced by fibrous tissue. In part these changes are due to deprivation of the normal activation by nerve impulses, but the more severe effects are attributable to the nerve degeneration and the consequent failure of what are called the trophic influences, which we can now ascribe to the macromolecular transport along the motor axons and across to the muscle fiber via the neuromuscular synapses, as generally indicated in Fig. 2-1*A*. We have no knowledge of these macromolecules,

B. Experiment as in *A*, but nerves were excised at 3 h, one being in a 2-mM solution of NaCN, the other in the normal moist chamber. Both were counted 6 h after the injection. (*From Ochs, 1972a.*)

but the transport has been found to be also fast, with an approximate speed of 360 mm/day. This measurement is derived from observations of Miledi and Slater showing that the onset of degenerative changes at the neuromuscular junction is more delayed the further the nerve section is from the muscle. The key role of macromolecular transport along the nerve fibers has now been demonstrated by the use of colchicine and vinblastin to block this transport. These substances break up the neuro-tubular system, but for some days do not prevent impulse propagation; nevertheless, the muscles display the excitability changes characteristic of denervated muscle.

In addition to this fast transport along nerve fibers, many other transport mechanisms have been described, some being almost as fast, but others much slower—at velocities measured in a few millimeters a day. There is need of much more experimental investigation, but in general it appears that there are three main modes of transportation along nerve fibers. The best investigated is the fast, as illustrated in Figs. 5-14 and 5-15. The slow tends to be about 100 times slower and moves soluble proteins and various structural proteins such as those depicted on the phospholipid membrane in Fig. 1-12. Finally, there is the reverse transport from axon to nerve cell. This retrograde transport can be seen in the movement of fine particles in cinemicroscopy. It is the basis of the remarkable technique of using *horseradish peroxidase* to identify the neurons sending axons to some particular site in the brain. The horserad-ish peroxidase is picked up by the axonal terminals and is retrogradely transported to their nerve cells in which characteristic structural changes are induced.

By radiotracer techniques Grafstein first demonstrated the trans-neuronal transport of labeled macromolecules from the injection site in the retina across the synapses in the lateral geniculate body and so to the visual cortex. This work has been dramatically confirmed by Wiesel and associates who have shown by autoradiography that from the injected eye there is a highly specific transport to the zones of the visual cortex that receive the visual input from the injected eye. Thus the path is selectively via the synapses of the lateral geniculate body (cf. Fig. 6-4*A*) and not diffusely by nonspecific channels. Transneuronal transport has been demonstrated in several other sites, and Cowan and Graybiel envisage the possibility that transsynaptic transport of macromolecules may be a generalized phenomenon in the brain.

General Summary

We can now conjecture that the whole nervous system has communica-tion not only by impulses that signal quickly in the manner described in the preceding chapters but also chemically by transport of specific proteins and other macromolecules. We can assume that this transport must go in the most incredibly complex manner between the neurons of the brain, organizing all their interrelationships in a way that we still cannot even imagine. We do know that, if a cell has most of the synapses on it degenerated, much like denervated muscle fibers, it dies too. This process is called *transneuronal degeneration.* Apparently a neuron does require the trophic transport from the synapses on it in order to keep alive, and this dependence goes on in turn from cell to cell to cell. Every cell, as it were, is talking chemically to all the other cells that it is connected with and instructing them how to talk to the next ones and so on. So this chemical manner of communication keeps the whole immense organized structure of the brain in some kind of dynamic state that we may call trophic resonance by this vast interlocking process of specific chemical communications. Here we are imagining far beyond experimental evidence, but such a vision is of the greatest value if it leads to the formulation of problems that can be experimentally attacked.

THE NEURONAL MECHANISM OF LEARNING AND MEMORY

Introduction

In this section I am concentrating on the neuronal machinery of the mammalian brain in order to reduce the subject to manageable proportions. I do not make detailed reference to the whole field of *conditioned reflexes.* My aim is to consider the neuronal mechanisms involved in all these learning and retrieval performances of the mammalian brain. Fortunately Kandel and Spencer have published a review that gives an excellent account of learning in the "brains" of invertebrates. It also gives a valuable review of the varieties of conditioned reflexes and of *habituation.*

Following Hebb, it is generally recognized that there are two kinds of learning and memory: *short-term* and *long-term.* However, we shall propose later that long-term memory is composed of an intermediate memory of hours and a truly long-term memory that can last for a lifetime. Short-term memory is exemplified in the ability to remember short sequences of digits, as for example a telephone number that you look up and then dial. If there are no special circumstances, the number sequence is lost in a few minutes beyond recall. This brief memory is most probably dependent on the patterned operations of neuronal circuits running in complex reentrant pathways in the cerebral cortex like those schematically illustrated in Fig. 6-6. These dots are nerve cells diagrammed in an assumed cluster arrangement (this will be described in the next chapter) with many lines in parallel, as in multilane traffic. It is assumed that, by their synaptic connections, impulses traverse neurons weaving a pattern in space and time that carries the information. This information can be retrieved by allowing the patterned operation to achieve expression. We may call it a *dynamic engram* to use Lashley's phrase for the neuronal basis of memory.

But this dynamic engram will not account for long-term memory because this memory is retained even after all neuronal activity in the cerebrum has been suppressed in coma, deep anesthesia, electroconvulsive shock, or extreme cold. For example, conditioned reflexes in animals and human memories survive these extreme treatments. So there must be some other neuronal mechanism for encoding long-term memories. It is postulated that this mechanism is based on some structural change that must be capable of being "read out" so that the code again gains expression in the neuronal operation of the brain. This is essentially Lashley's concept of the engram.

Synaptic Plasticity and Learning

In general terms we have to consider that long-term memories are somehow encoded in the neuronal connectivities of the brain. We are thus led to postulate that the structural basis lies in modifications of synapses. In mammals there is no evidence for growth or change of neuronal pathways in the brain after their initial formation. It is not possible to construct or reconstruct brain pathways at such a gross level. But it should be possible to secure the necessary plastic changes in neuronal connectivity by microstructural changes in synapses. For example, they may be hypertrophied or they may bud additional synapses, or alternatively they may regress. Since it would be expected that this increased synaptic efficacy would arise because of strong synaptic activation, experiments such as those illustrated in Fig. 5-16 have been carried out on many types of synapses.

Figure 5-16*A* and *B* is remarkable in showing that repetitive stimulation results in a large increase (up to 6 times) in the EPSPs monosynaptically produced in an α motoneuron by pyramidal tract fibers (cf. Figs. 4-2 and 4-7), whereas the monosynaptic EPSPs by the Ia fibers on that same motoneuron (cf Fig. 3-2) were not potentiated. Evidently the pyramidal tract synapses display an extreme range of modifiability by what we may call *frequency potentiation*. The synaptic mechanism involved in this potentiation is not understood, but we can be sure that it is due to an equivalent increase in emission of transmitter. Many types of synapses at the higher levels of the brain have this ability to build up operationally during intense activation.

The series of Fig. 5-16*C* and *D* gives another example for synapses in a primitive part of the cerebrum, the hippocampus. Part *D* shows the

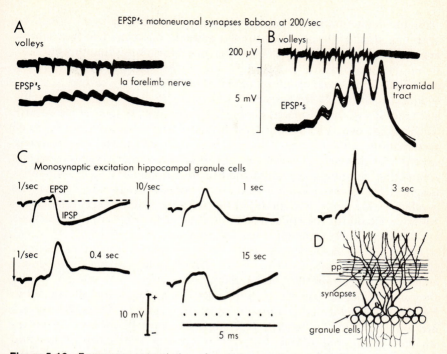

Figure 5-16 Frequency potentiation of excitatory synapses. *A,B.* The lower traces are monosynaptic EPSPs of the same motoneuron of the cervical enlargement of the baboon spinal cord, there being in each case six stimuli at 200 per second to the Ia afferent pathway in *A* and to the pyramidal tract in *B.* [*S. Landgren, C. G. Phillips, and R. Porter, J. Physiol.,* **161**:91 (1962).] *C* shows frequency potentiation of monosynaptic EPSPs of hippocampal granule cells when the frequency of stimulation of the perforating pathway (pp of D) was increased from 1 to 10 per s, and its decline on return to 1 per s.. (*From Lomo, 1970.*)

excitatory synapses from the perforating pathway (pp) onto the dendrites of the granule cells. In *C* the intracellular record from a granule cell during the initial series at 1 per s stimulation of pp showed a very small initial EPSP followed by a large IPSP. With the stimulus frequency raised to 10 per s, already within 1 s there was a large potentiation of the EPSP that counteracted to some extent the IPSP. After 3 s of this stimulation the very large EPSP is seen to generate an impulse discharge from the cell. On again slowing the stimulation to 1 per s, the frequency potentiation had already considerably declined at 0.4 s and had disappeared in 15 s. It is attractive to think that synapses responding as enthusiastically to intense activation could be the *modifiable synapses* responsible for the phenomena of learning and memory.

Although this synaptic potentiation during stimulation is of interest in relationship to the synaptic modification required for learning, any prolonged potentiation after the intense synaptic activation would be nearer to a possible paradigm of the learning process. This *posttetanic potentiation* has been very fully investigated for monosynaptic action on spinal motoneurons (cf. Fig. 3-2). In Fig. 5-17*A* and *B* the intracellularly recorded EPSPs were almost doubled in size after severe synaptic activations (640 per s for 5 s, and 640 per s for 30 s), as may be seen in the inset records of the EPSPs at the height of potentiation and of the control EPSPs. However, the plotted points in *A* and *B* show that all trace of potentiation had disappeared in a few minutes. Even after an extremely severe stimulation in *C* (500 per s for 20 min—600,000 impulses) the posttetanic potentiation had declined to zero in just over 2 h. Evidently, the synapses in the spinal cord exhibit no indefinitely prolonged increase in efficacy that could be a model of the learning process. This failure was not unexpected for the spinal cord, for at this level of the central nervous system there is no good evidence for memory.

Figure 5-18 shows a remarkably different kind of posttetanic potentiation in the hippocampus, which is a special type of cerebral cortex that is believed to be important in memory. Frequency potentiation of the excitatory synapses on the granule cells has already been illustrated in Fig. 5-16*C*. A very mild stimulation of 20 per s for 15 s (300 impulses) was applied at the first arrow. The plotted points show that there was only a small transient potentiation. But, with successive repetitions of this mild stimulation about every half hour, there was a progressive increase in the potentiation so that after the fifth there was an enormous potentiation of the impulse discharge from the granule cells. Actual records are given in the insets, where three test responses may be compared with three controls given by the other side. The plotted measurements are of the sharp downward extracellular spike. This large potentiation continued for 3 h. This amazing effect was regularly observed in many such experiments, potentiations being fully maintained even for 10 h. We can conclude that in these experiments Lømo and associates have demonstrated that the synapses on the hippocampal granule cells are modifiable to a high degree and exhibit a prolonged potentiation that could be the physiological expression of the memory process.

Physiological experiments have indicated that the modifiable synapses that could be responsible for memory are excitatory and are specially prominent at the higher levels of the brain. In the cerebral cortex the great majority of excitatory synapses on pyramidal cells are on their dendritic spines, as illustrated in Figs. 1-3*B*, 3-14, and 4-6. There is also much evidence that these spine synapses regress during disuse. Hence, it is postulated that these spine synapses on the dendrites of such neurons as the pyramidal cells of the cerebral cortex and the Purkinje cells of the cerebellum are the modifiable synapses concerned in learning. These would be the synapses displaying the indefinitely prolonged potentiation

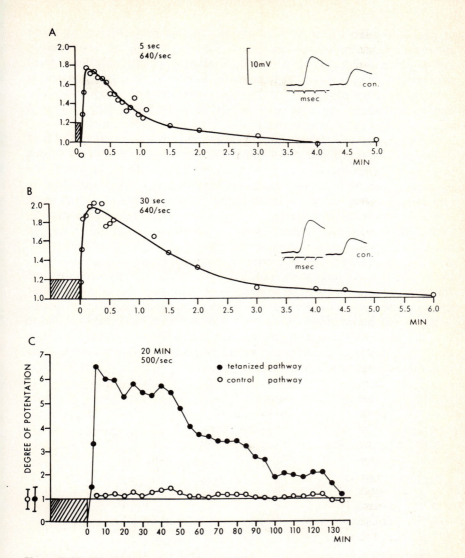

Figure 5-17 Posttetanic potentiation of EPSPs generated by Ia synapses on motoneu-rons. *A,B.* The conditioning tetani are specified and also are indicated by the cross-hatched rectangles. The plotted points give the ratio of the potentiated EPSPs to the initial control at the indicated intervals after the end of the tetanus. Further description in text. [*D. R. Curtis and J. C. Eccles, J. Physiol.,* **150:**374 *(1960).*] In *C* there was a much more severe conditioning tetanus. The plotted filled circles show the monosynaptic reflex discharges observed in the ventral root at up to 135 min after the end of the tetanus and calculated relative to the initial control reflex, each plotted point being the mean of 10 to 20 individual responses. The open circles are for similar responses recorded on the contralateral unstimulated side and serve to monitor the general level of reflex activity during the experiment. (*From Spencer; illustrated in Kandel and Spencer, 1968.*)

of Fig. 5-18. One can imagine that the superior performance by these synapses was so prolonged because a growth process had developed in the dendritic spines giving a structural change which could have great endurance. There is as yet no convincing demonstration of this growth in electron micrographs, but there is much circumstantial evidence. The expected changes are diagrammatically shown in Fig. 5-19, where *A* represents the normal state and *B* and *C* the potentiated states.

We are on much surer histological grounds in showing the effects of disuse in causing a depletion of spine synapses (Fig. 5-19*D*), because this has been beautifully demonstrated by Valverde on the dendrites of the pyramidal cells in the visual cortex of mice raised in visual deprivation, and indeed similar demonstrations have been made with other spine synapses. So it can be assumed that normal usage results in the maintenance of the dendritic spine synapses at the level of Fig. 5-19*A*. An alternative to the synaptic spine hypertrophy of Fig. 5-19*B* is shown in *C* where an increase in synaptic potency has been secured by branching of the spines to form secondary spine synapses as reported by Szentágothai. It can be concluded that the spine synapses are probably the modifiable synapses concerned in memory, but much more rigid experimental testing with systematic electron microscopic examination is urgently needed to test this hypothesis. It is surprising that there has as yet been no such systematic study of synapses in the hippocampus under conditions that would be expected to show synaptic hypertrophy.

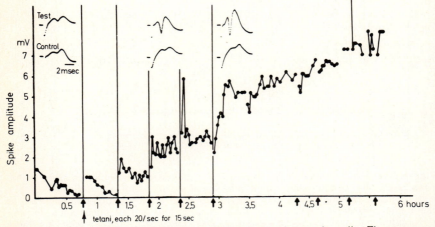

Figure 5-18 Posttetanic potentiation of hippocampal granule cells. The measurements were made on the extracellular recording of the positive spike shown in the specimen records, and it may be taken to be a measure of the number of granule cells firing impulses in the zone sampled by the recording electrode. Further description in text. [*T. V. A. Bliss and T. Lømo, J. Physiol.,* **232**:*331 (1973) and personal communication.*]

This simple concept that disuse leads to regression of spine synapses and excess usage to hypertrophy can be criticized because it is now recognized that almost all cells at the highest levels of the nervous system are discharging impulses continuously (cf. Figs. 4-4 and 4-19). One can imagine therefore that there would be overall hypertrophy of all synapses under such conditions of continued activation, and hence but little possibility of any selective hypertrophic change. Evidently, frequent synaptic excitation alone could hardly provide a satisfactory explanation of synaptic changes involved in learning. Such "learned" synapses would be too ubiquitous! This criticism of the simple *"growth theory"* of learning can perhaps be contained by the recent suggestions of Szentágothai and Marr that synaptic learning is a dual or dynamically linked happening, namely that activation of a special type of synapse provides instructions for the growth of other activated synapses on the same dendrite. This may be called the *"conjunction theory of learning."* It was originally suggested that the unique operation of climbing fibers on the Purkinje dendrites of the cerebellum (Fig. 4-11) was to give "growth instructions" to the spine synapses that are simultaneously activated by the parallel fibers. It is as if the climbing-fiber impulses said: "Now learn!" and that otherwise activation of the spine synapses did not result in growth and the long-term memory encoded thereby.

By most ingenious experiments Ito and associates have provided the first evidence in favor of the conjunction theory of learning. When animals are rotated on a vertical axis, mossy-fiber and climbing-fiber inputs to a special lobe of the cerebellum (the flocculus) are concerned in controlling the eye movements so that the visual picture suffers a minimum of disturbance. When climbing-fiber input from the visual pathways is superimposed on the mossy-fiber input from the vestibular

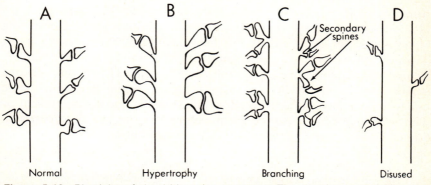

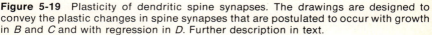

Figure 5-19 Plasticity of dendritic spine synapses. The drawings are designed to convey the plastic changes in spine synapses that are postulated to occur with growth in *B* and *C* and with regression in *D*. Further description in text.

pathway, a plastic change results so that the vestibular input becomes more effective in the control of the eye movements. It appears that the climbing-fiber input has resulted in the Purkinje cells learning to respond more effectively to the mossy-fiber input. In a complementary investigation Hámori has produced anatomical evidence that in cats the climbing-fiber synapses on Purkinje cells exert a trophic influence causing the Purkinje dendrites to generate spines that are the synaptic sites for the mossy-fiber pathway via parallel fibers (cf. Fig. 4-11). Kawaguchi has demonstrated in kittens a remarkable trophic influence of climbing fibers in causing the profuse branching of the dendritic trees of Purkinje cells (cf. Fig. 4-11). Sotelo and associates report in rats contrary findings to those of Hámori and Kawaguchi in cats. A species difference seems to be indicated.

Much more complicated neuronal systems are concerned in the establishment of long-term memories in the cerebral cortex, but in essentials there is a remarkable operation of a conjunction mechanism. Circuits from the parietal, temporal, and frontal lobes through the hippocampus play a key role, but there are many other structures associated with this hippocampal circuit from and to the neocortex. In addition there are reverberatory circuits from the hippocampus to other limbic structures, as described by Kornhuber. The essential role of these circuits in the *consolidation of a memory trace* (as it is called) is dramatically shown by the tragic disability of a patient suffering from bilateral destruction of the hippocampus and/or associated structures on these postulated looping circuits. There is an almost complete failure to establish memories for any happenings or experiences after the occurrence of the lesion. The patient with this *amnestic syndrome*, as it is called, lives entirely with short-term memories of a few seconds duration and with the memories retained from before the lesion. It is important to recognize that the hippocampus is not the seat of the memory stores. Memories from before the lesion are well retained and recalled. The hippocampal system is merely the instrument responsible for the laying down of the memory trace or engram, which presumably is very largely located in the neocortex in the appropriate areas. There is no obvious impairment of personality in these patients despite the catastrophic failure of memory. In fact they live either in the immediate present or with remembered experience from before the time of the operation. Milner gives a graphic account of a patient with the amnestic syndrome:

His mother observes that he will do the same jigsaw puzzle day after day without showing any practice effect, and read the same magazines over and over again without finding their contents familiar. The same forgetfulness applies to people he has met since the lesion, even to those neighbors who have been visiting the house regularly for the past six years. He has not learned their names and he does not recognize any of them if he meets them in the street.

In summary of the hippocampal role in memory it can be stated that: (1) In retrieving the memory of an event that is not being continuously rehearsed in the short-term memory process, the self-conscious mind is dependent on some consolidation or storage process that is brought about by hippocampal activity; (2) the hippocampus and associated structures are not the site of the storage; (3) we conjecture that the hippocampal participation in the consolidation process is dependent on neural pathways that transmit from the neocortex to the hippocampal complex and thence back to the neocortex, there being several synaptic relays in each stage of the circuit. The effectiveness of this circuit probably depends on its repetitive activity in some closed-loop manner. Figures 5-16 and 5-18 illustrate the amazing ability of the hippocampal granule cells to increase in their synaptic responsiveness during and after repetitive activation. We can conjecture that the hippocampal circuits act on the neocortical synapses in an instructional manner.

If synaptic growth is required for learning, there must be an increase in brain metabolism of a special kind with the manufacture of proteins and other macromolecules required for the membranes and the chemical transmission mechanism (cf. Figs. 1-12, 2-10, and 2-11). In neurochemistry and neuropharmacology there have now been many fine studies by Barondes, Agranoff, and others, which reveal that long-term learning does not occur when either cerebral protein synthesis or RNA synthesis is greatly depressed by enzyme poisons. It is suggested that, in the process of learning, neuronal activation leads first to specific RNA synthesis and this in turn to protein synthesis and so finally to synaptic growth and the encoding of the memory. The approximate time of about 30 minutes to 3 hours seems to be required for the synaptic growth giving long-term memory. There must be an *intermediate-term memory* to bridge the gap between the short-term memory of seconds and the onset of the synaptic growth giving true long-term memory. It is suggested that the posttetanic potentiation illustrated in Figs. 5-17 and 5-18 is exactly fitted for providing the intermediate-term memory. It would be induced by the repetitive synaptic activations of short-term memory and would immediately follow those actions, being restricted to the activated synapses and being graded in accord with their action. It has to be recognized that intermediate-term memory is also dependent on the hippocampal circuits. It is therefore of importance that in Fig. 5-18 posttetanic potentiation enduring for hours followed quite mild repetitive stimulation of hippocampal synapses.

There is thus ample overlap between this postulated intermediate-term memory and the metabolically induced growth that provides the enduring base for true long-term memory.

Libet and associates have very recently proposed a model for a synaptic memory process that is also a conjunction process between two different synapses on a sympathetic ganglion cell: "A heterosynaptic interaction takes place between two types of synaptic inputs to the same neurone; the memory trace is initiated by a brief (dopaminergic) input in one synaptic line, while 'read-out' of the memory consists simply in the enhanced ability of the postsynaptic unit to produce its specific response to another (cholinergic) synaptic input. This arrangement provides for a 'learned' change in the response to one input as a result of an 'experience' previously carried by way of the other input." This model is based on carefully controlled responses of sympathetic ganglion cells, which display a doubling of response to acetylcholine for many hours after a brief exposure to the other transmitter, dopamine. Furthermore it is shown that cyclic AMP is concerned in the metabolic pathway that gives the heterosynaptic potentiation. It is evident that this discovery is of great significance in relation to the conjunction theory of learning.

The Engram as a Basis of Learning and Retrieval (Memory)

Let us now return to consider how synaptic hypertrophy could be the structural basis of long-term memory. We may regard Fig. 6-6 as giving a greatly simplified picture of the way in which unique spatiotemporal patterns may be generated by the sequential firing of neurons in complex circuits in the brain. It is a general postulate of brain action that conscious experiences derive from some of these complex patterned performances, the uniqueness of the pattern matching the uniqueness of the experience derived therefrom. If it so happens that a spatiotemporal pattern of neuronal activation is an approximate copy of that played on an earlier occasion, the subject will derive an experience that he recognizes as a remembrance of that experience which was of course derived from the original of the copy. We have to imagine that in the brain there are immense numbers of patterns (engrams) encoded in the neuronal connectivities established by selective synaptic hypertrophies in the way I have described. When activated, these patterns of connectivity result in spatiotemporal patterns of impulses that are approximate copies of the patterns responsible for the original experience and are available for readout and hence for memory retrieval. Thus there are in the brain, and particularly in the cerebral cortex, these immense numbers of patterns of specific neuronal connectivities (engrams) ready for replay so that impulse patterns can arise that are approximate copies of those involved in the original experience. You will appreciate that the most bothersome problem about memory is to effect retrieval on demand. It can be thought of as the problem of initiating the replay of the engram. I myself have to use a whole repertoire of tricks and subterfuges to gain "entry" to many of my engrams. Expressed in neural terms, I have to be able to "trigger" the whole patterned replay by some initiating neural input. My problem is to be able to conjure up the effective input, and all this is required merely to remember a name, for example.

Now you might say this engram concept is asking too much—one experience, just one accident, for example, just for a moment, sudden, intense—how can it produce a stabilized brain change, an engram, so that you can remember it all your life? But in my experience these striking remembered events are reexperienced to a fantastic degree. We can all recall such happenings that we cannot get out of our mind for days. When you have had some intense, tragic, or exciting experience, it is later replayed again and again in the neuronal mechanisms of your brain. The more you replay, the more the activated synapses can be assumed to hypertrophy and stabilize the neural pathways, and so the more vivid and enduring is the memory.

I believe that this general concept leads to some understanding of how the brain can remember. It is the replaying of neuronal pathways that have become effective operationally because of the initial intense synaptic activations. The pathway is given a potential stability as an engram because its constituent synapses have grown to be bigger and better. There is no construction of large new pathways, such as could happen with fish and amphibia, but just microstructural changes, slightly bigger synaptic knobs or branching knobs such as are illustrated in Fig. 5-19*B* and *C*.

GENERAL CONCLUSIONS

In the preceding chapters I have dealt with elementary levels of brain operation, taking the brain and its constituent neurons as given. At all levels the responses of the brain have been explained as being due to transmission by nerve impulses. The input from receptor organs via synaptic action and the many sequential synaptic relays lead eventually to the discharge of motoneurons, with the ensuing muscle contractions giving movement. At the higher levels of the brain the neuronal pathways are of immense complexity, and in principle it can be conceived that these pathways provide an adequate explanation of even the most complex and subtle human performances. This claim provides the theme for discussion in Chap. 6. Yet many problems remain, even if this program were successful in identifying all brain responses as being due to the operations of what we may call its constituent neuronal machinery.

First, we have the immense problem of the building of the brain with all the lines of communication in pathways that have detailed topographic relations. In this chapter we have seen that this turns out to be a problem of genetic instructions that achieve expression as specific molecular labels on the individual neurons. But neurons are not isolated entities. They develop together with their chemical sensing and recognition and there are many indications that this specific chemical communication continues throughout life. It is important to recognize that the neurons of the brain are not only linked by impulse communication but also by special chemical transmission such as is displayed in the trophic reactions.

Second, the brain is not a fixed action structure. At the higher levels of the brain, modifiability is the essence of its performance, as is evidenced by learning and memory. We have seen that this could be explained by microstructural changes. It is postulated that synaptic activity leads to their growth by its effect in causing the synthesis of RNA and so of the enzymes building proteins and other macromolecules. Palay can now distinguish, in electron micrographs of the brain, synapses in various stages of growth and dissolution, and comparable observations have been made by Barker and associates on the neuromuscular synapses. In contrast to the commonly accepted belief of a static structure, we have to think of the brain as being structurally plastic at the microlevel— some synapses being mature, others developing, others regressing.

Finally, it should be noted that the brain is composed of glial cells as well as neurons. The glia have been neglected in this account of the brain which has been concentrated on the neuronal mechanisms and impulse transmission. The investigations of Kuffler and his associates have now established that glia are not concerned in impulse transmission, but function in metabolic relationship with neurons, in guiding their growth and possibly in limiting ion accumulation in the extracellular spaces. I like to think of them as the "housemaids" of the brain, being particularly concerned in the transport of materials from the blood vessels to the neurons and vice versa. They fulfill an important role not only in the nutrition of the brain but also in its protection against poisons by contributing to the so-called blood-brain barrier.

REFERENCES

Altman, J. (1972a): "Postnatal Development of the Cerebellar Cortex in the Rat: I. The External Germinal Layer and the Transitional Molecular Layer," *J. Comp. Neur.*, **145**:353–398.
Altman, J. (1972b): "Postnatal Development of the Cerebellar Cortex in the Rat: II. Phases in the Maturation of Purkinje Cells and of the Molecular Layer," *J. Comp. Neur.*, **145**:399–464.

Altman, J. (1972c): "Postnatal Development of the Cerebellar Cortex in the Rat: III. Maturation of the Components of the Granular Layer," *J. Comp. Neur.*, **145:**465–514.

Barondes, S. H. (1967): "Axoplasmic Transport," *Neurosci. Res. Progr. Bull.*, **5:**307–419.

Barondes, S. H. (1970): "Multiple Steps in the Biology of Memory," in F. O. Schmitt (ed.), *The Neurosciences*, Rockefeller University Press, New York, pp. 272–278.

Brodal, A. (1973): "Self-Observations and Neuro-Anatomical Considerations after a Stroke," *Brain*, **96:**675–694.

Buller, A. J. (1972): "The Neural Control of Some Characteristics of Skeletal Muscle," in C. B. B. Downman (ed.), *Modern Trends in Physiology*, Butterworth, London, pp. 72–85.

Buller, A. J., W. F. H. M. Mommaerts, and K. Seraydarian (1969): "Enzymic Properties of Myosin in Fast and Slow Twitch Muscles of the Cat Following Cross-Innervation," *J. Physiol.*, **205:**581–597.

Cowan, W. M. (1971): "Studies on the Development of the Avian Visual System," in D. S. Pease (ed.), *Cellular Aspects of Neural Growth and Differentiation*, University of California Press, Los Angeles, pp. 177–218.

Eccles, J. C. (1958): "Problems of Plasticity and Organization at Simplest Levels of Mammalian Central Nervous System," *Perspectives Biol. Med.*, **1:**379–396.

Eccles, J. C. (1967): "The Effects of Nerve Cross Union on Muscle Contraction," in A. T. Milhorat (ed.), *Exploratory Concepts in Muscular Dystrophy and Related Disorders*, Excerpta Medica Foundation, Amsterdam, pp. 151–160.

Eccles, J. C. (1970): "Neurogenesis and Morphogenesis in the Cerebellar Cortex," *Proc. Nat. Acad. Sci. U.S.*, **66:**294–301.

Eccles, J. C. (1972): "Possible Synaptic Mechanisms Subserving Learning," in A. G. Karczmar and J. C. Eccles (eds.), *Brain and Human Behavior*, Springer, Heidelberg.

Eccles, J. C. (1974): "Trophic Interactions in the Mammalian Central Nervous System," in D. B. Drachman (ed.), *Trophic Functions of the Neuron*, Ann. N.Y. Acad. Sci., **228:**406–422.

Eccles, J. C. (1976): "The Plasticity of the Mammalian Central Nervous System with Special Reference to New Growths in Response to Lesions," *Naturwissenschaften*, **63:**8–15.

Edds, Mac V., D. S. Barkley, and D. M. Fambrough (1972): "Genesis of Neuronal Patterns," *Neurosci. Res. Progr. Bull.*, **10:**253–367.

Gaze, R. M. (1970): *The Formation of Nerve Connections*, Academic Press, London and New York.

Grafstein, B. (1971): "Transneuronal Transfer of Radioactivity in the Central Nervous System," *Science*, **172:**177–179.

Graybiel, A. M. (1976): "Wallerian Degeneration and Anterograde Tracer Methods," (in course of publication).

Guth, L. (1968): " 'Trophic' Influences of Nerve on Muscle," *Physiol. Rev.*, **48:**645–687.

Hámori, J. (1972): "Developmental Morphology of Dendritic Postsynaptic Specializations," in K. Lissák (ed.), *Recent Development of Neurobiology in Hungary*, vol. 4, Akademia Kiado, Budapest, pp. 9–32.

Hebb, D. O. (1949): *The Organization of Behaviour*, Wiley, New York.

Jacobson, M. (1970): *Developmental Neurobiology*, Holt, Rinehart & Winston, New York.

Kandel, E. R., and W. A. Spencer (1968): "Cellular Neurophysiological Approaches in the Study of Learning," *Physiol. Rev.*, **48**:65–134.

Kornhuber, H. H. (1975): "Neuronal Control of Input into Long Term Memory: Limbic System and Amnestic Syndrome in Man," in H. P. Zippel (ed.), *Memory and Transfer of Information*, Plenum, New York.

Kuffler, S. W. (1966): "Physiological Properties of Vertebrate and Invertebrate Neuroglial Cells and the Movement of Substances through the Nervous System," *Proc. Roy. Soc. B*, **168**:1–21.

Lashley, K. S. (1950): "In Search of the Engram," *Symp. Soc. Exp. Biol.*, **4**:454–482.

Libet, B., H. Kobayashi, and T. Tanaka (1975): "Synaptic Coupling into the Production and Storage of a Memory Trace." *Nature* **258**:155–157.

Lømo, T. (1970): "Some Properties of a Cortical Excitatory Synapse," in P. Andersen and J. K. S. Jansen (eds.), *Excitatory Synaptic Mechanisms*, Universitetsforlaget, Oslo, pp. 207–211.

Miledi, R., and C. R. Slater (1970): "On the Degeneration of Rat Neuromuscular Junctions After Nerve Section," *J. Physiol.*, **207**:507–528.

Milner, B. (1966): "Amnesia following Operation on the Temporal Lobes," in C. W. M. Whitty and O. L. Zangwill (eds.), *Amnesia*, Butterworths, London, pp. 109–133.

Milner, B. (1970): "Memory and the Medial Temporal Regions of the Brain," in K. H. Pribram and D. E. Broadbent (eds.), *Biology of Memory*, Academic Press, New York and London, pp. 29–50.

Mugnaini, E. (1970): "Neurones as Synaptic Targets," in P. Andersen and J. K. S. Jansen (eds.), *Excitatory Synaptic Mechanisms*, Universitetsforlaget, Oslo, pp. 149–169.

Ochs, S. (1972a): "The Dependence of Fast Transport in Mammalian Nerve Fibers on Metabolism," *Acta Neuropath.* (suppl.), **5**:86–96.

Ochs, S. (1972b): "Fast Transport of Materials in Mammalian Nerve Fibers," *Science*, **176**:252–260.

Raisman, G., and P. M. Field (1973): "A Quantitative Investigation of the Development of Collateral Reinnervation after Partial Deafferentation of the Septal Nuclei," *Brain Res.*, **50**:241–264.

Ramón y Cajal, S. (1960): *Studies on Vertebrate Neurogenesis.*, L. Guth (transl.), Charles C. Thomas, Springfield, Ill.

Sperry, R. W. (1951a): "Mechanisms of Neural Maturation," in S. S. Stevens (ed.), *Handbook of Experimental Psychology*, Wiley, New York.

Sperry, R. W. (1951b): "Regulative Factors in the Orderly Growth of Neural Circuits," *Growth Symp.*, **10**:63–87.

Sperry, R. W. (1956): "The Eye and the Brain," *Sci. Amer.*, **194**:48–52.

Sperry, R. W. (1959): "The Growth of Nerve Circuits," *Sci. Amer.*; reprinted in *From Cell to Organism*, Freeman, San Francisco, 1967, pp. 186–193.

Sperry, R. W. (1963): "Chemoaffinity in the Orderly Growth of Nerve Fiber Patterns and Connections," *Proc. Nat. Acad. Sci. U.S.*, **50**:703–710.

Sperry, R. W. (1971): "How a Developing Brain Gets Itself Properly Wired for Adaptive Function," in *Biopsychology of Development*, Academic Press, New York, pp. 27–44.

Szentágothai, J. (1971): "Memory Functions and the Structural Organization of the Brain," *Symposia Biologica Hungarica*, **10**:21–35.

Weiss, P. (1960): "The Concept of Perpetual Neuronal Growth and Proximo-Distal Substance Convection," in *4th Int. Neurochem. Symp.*, Pergamon, Oxford, pp. 220–242.

Wiesel, T. N., D. H. Hubel, and D. M. K. Lam (1974): "Autoradiographic Demonstration by Ocular-Dominance Columns in the Monkey Striate Cortex by Means of Transneuronal Transport," *Brain Res.*, **79**:273–279.

Yoon, M. G. (1975): "On Topographic Polarity of the Optic Tectum in Goldfish," in *The Synapse*, Cold Spring Harbor Symp. Quant. Biol., vol. 40.

Chapter 6

Brain, Speech, and Consciousness

In this chapter I have set myself an immense task. Let us look again at the brain as it can be seen in Fig. 4-1, located inside the skull. It has various specific areas marked on it. In Chap. 4 there was reference to the motor cortex which is the departure area for nerve impulses passing down the pyramidal tract eventually to bring about movement, and just behind it is the sensory area which is the impulse-arrival area from the whole body. Likewise on this brain it is shown that visual impressions arrive at the occipital lobe and auditory input at the upper part of the temporal lobe. These various areas are not responsible for perceptual recognition, but are merely the arrival and departure stations on the way into and out from the immensely complex neuronal machinery of the cortex. In Fig. 6-8 there are shown the speech areas that will be our especial concern in this chapter. There is a large area on the left temporoparietal lobe of the brain and another area in the inferior frontal lobe and also a small supplementary area. These areas are only in one hemisphere, which is almost always the left (98 percent). The right hemisphere (Fig. 6-9) is the same for motor and sensory function, but there are no areas specifically associated with speech.

We have to try and peer in depth through the substance of the brain and see how it can give us all the richness and variety of conscious experience. We can define problems in relation to the higher functions of the brain and I believe that we can look with new eyes at this whole story because of remarkable recent discoveries I will refer to later.

PHILOSOPHIC INTRODUCTION

Now before discussing brain function in detail I will at the beginning give an account of my philosophical position on the so-called *brain-mind problem* so that you will be able to relate the experimental evidence to this philosophical position. I have written at length on this philosophy in my book *Facing Reality* and more recently in a book with Sir Karl Popper, entitled *The Self and Its Brain*. In Fig. 6-1 you will be able to see that I fully accept the philosophical achievements of Sir Karl Popper with his concept of three worlds. I was a dualist, now I am a *trialist!* Cartesian dualism has become unfashionable with many people. They embrace monism in order to escape the enigma of brain-mind interaction with its perplexing problems. But Sir Karl Popper and I are interactionists, and what is more, *trialist interactionists*. The three worlds are very easily defined. I believe that in the classification of Fig. 6-1 there is nothing left out. It takes care of everything that is in existence and in our experience. All can be classified in one or other of the categories enumerated under Worlds 1, 2, and 3.

The Nature of Worlds 1, 2, and 3

In Fig. 6-1, World 1 is the world of physical objects and states. It comprises the whole cosmos of matter and energy, all of biology including

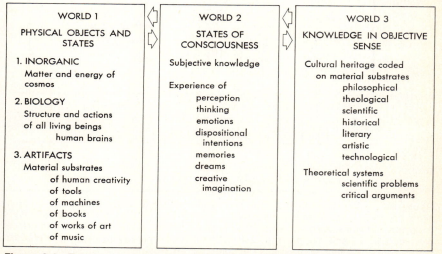

WORLD 1	WORLD 2	WORLD 3
PHYSICAL OBJECTS AND STATES	STATES OF CONSCIOUSNESS	KNOWLEDGE IN OBJECTIVE SENSE
1. INORGANIC Matter and energy of cosmos 2. BIOLOGY Structure and actions of all living beings human brains 3. ARTIFACTS Material substrates of human creativity of tools of machines of books of works of art of music	Subjective knowledge Experience of perception thinking emotions dispositional intentions memories dreams creative imagination	Cultural heritage coded on material substrates philosophical theological scientific historical literary artistic technological Theoretical systems scientific problems critical arguments

Figure 6-1 Tabular representation of the three worlds that comprise all existences and all experiences as defined by Popper (1972). (*From Eccles, 1970.*)

human brains, and all artifacts that man has made for coding information, as for example the paper and ink of books or the material base of works of art. World 1 is the total world of the materialists. They recognize nothing else. All else is fantasy.

World 2 is the world of states of consciousness and subjective knowledge of all kinds. The totality of our perceptions comes in this world. But there are several levels. In agreement with Polten, I tend to recognize three kinds of levels of World 2, as indicated in Fig. 6-2, but it may be more correct to think of it as a spectrum.

The first level (*outer sense*) would be the ordinary perceptions provided by all our sense organs, hearing and touch and sight and smell and pain. All of these perceptions are in World 2, of course: vision with light and color; sound with music and harmony; touch with all its qualities and vibration; the range of odors and tastes, and so on. These qualities do not exist in World 1, where correspondingly there are but electromagnetic waves, pressure waves in the atmosphere, material objects, and chemical substances.

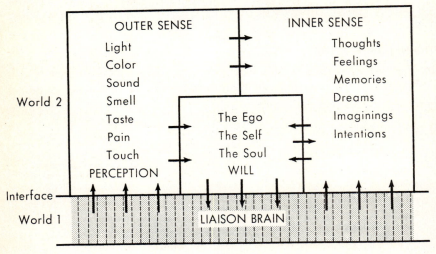

BRAIN⇌MIND INTERACTION

Figure 6-2 Information flow diagram for brain-mind interaction. The three components of World 2: outer sense, inner sense, and the ego (or self) are diagrammed with their connectivities. Also shown are the lines of communication across the interface between World 1 and World 2, that is, from the liaison brain to and from these World 2 components. The liaison brain has the columnar arrangement indicated (cf. Figs. 4-5, 4-6, 6-5). It must be imagined that the area of the liaison brain is enormous with open modules or columns numbering a hundred thousand or more, not just the two score here depicted.

In addition there is a level of *inner sense*, which is the world of more subtle perceptions. It is the world of your emotions, of your feelings of joy and sadness and fear and anger and so on. It includes all your memory, and all your imaginings and planning into the future. In fact there is a whole range of levels which could be described at length. All the subtle experiences of the human person are in this inner sensory world. It is all private to you but you can reveal it in linguistic expression, and by gestures of all levels of subtlety.

Finally, at the core of World 2 there is the *self* or *ego*, which is the basis of our unity as an experiencing being throughout our whole lifetime.

This World 2 is our *primary reality*. Our conscious experiences are the basis of our knowledge of World 1, which is thus a world of *secondary reality*, a derivative world. Whenever I am doing a scientific experiment, for example, I have to plan it cognitively, all in my thoughts, and then consciously carry out my plan of action in the experiment. Finally I have to look at the results and evaluate them in thought. For example, I have to see the traces on the oscilloscope and their photographic records or hear the signals on the loudspeaker. The various signals from the recording equipment have to be received by my sense organs, transmitted to my brain, and so to my consciousness, then appropriately measured and compared before I can begin to think about the significance of the experimental results. We are all the time, in every action we do, incessantly playing backwards and forwards between World 1 and World 2.

And what is World 3? As shown in Fig. 6-1 it is the whole world of culture. It is the world that was created by man and that reciprocally made man. This is my message in which I follow Popper unreservedly. The whole of language is here. All our means of communication, all our intellectual efforts coded in books, coded in the artistic and technological treasures in the museums, coded in every artifact left by man from primitive times—this is World 3 right up to the present time. It is the world of civilization and culture. Education is the means whereby each human being is brought into relation with World 3. In this manner he becomes immersed in it throughout life, participating in the heritage of mankind and so becoming fully human. World 3 is the world that uniquely relates to man. It is the world which is completely unknown to animals. They are blind to all of World 3. I say that without any reservations. This is then the first part of my story.

Interaction of Worlds 1, 2, and 3

Now I come to consider the way in which the three worlds interact. Figure 6-3 is a representation of lines of communication. It is not an anatomical diagram. The brain is enlarged and the body attenuated because it is not directly concerned in the communication, and both are shown to be in World 1. Arrows indicate the pathways from the sense organs to the brain (Aff. path) and the pathways out from the brain by nerves to muscles (Eff. path).

Following Sherrington in his great book *Man on his Nature*, I postulated many years ago in my book *The Neurophysiological Basis of*

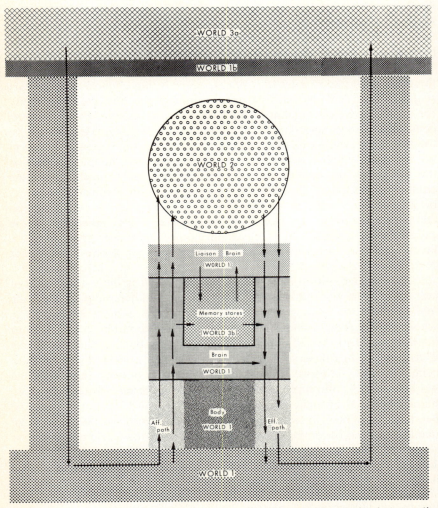

Figure 6-3 Information flow diagram representing modes of interaction between the three worlds as shown by the pathways represented by arrows. It is to be noted that, except for the liaison between the brain (World 1) and World 2 all of the information flow is in the matter-energy system of World 1. Further description in text. (*From Eccles, 1970.*)

Mind that there was a part of the brain, the *liaison brain*, in which special kinds of activity gave you conscious experience. For many years this concept of a special liaison brain has been left aside—neglected or rejected—but now it is being more favorably considered because it is even possible to give it an approximate anatomical location and to define it in a way that could not have been predicted. This liaison brain diagrammed in Fig. 6-3 and the spatiotemporal pattern of impulses in it are the necessary conditions for perceptions in World 2. For example, on the cognitive side, brain actions which we will consider later give experiences and these experiences can result in thoughts that lead to a disposition to do something and so to the operation of free will—of thought taking expression in action.

In Fig. 6-3 World 3 is shown symbolically spreading indefinitely across the top of the diagram. It represents the whole of culture but of course it has to be coded on World 1 materials (shown as World 1b), e.g., the paper and ink of books. And World 3 can only be experienced in World 2 by a complex pathway through World 1. For example, in order to read a book illumination is essential, then in an appropriate manner the radiation from the printed page is focused into an image on the retina and so, by coding into nerve impulses, it is transmitted to the visual cortex. Here there begin processes of decoding that eventually in the linguistic and liaison areas are transformed into neuronal patterns that appear in World 2 (note upward arrows) as meaningful sentences and result cognitively as some understanding or emotional feeling or aesthetic appreciation for example. These vague statements are the best that we can make on this wonderful process of extracting thoughts from the printed page, as I hope you are doing now.

In each of us there is a continuous and intense interaction and flow between the three worlds of Fig. 6-3. World 1 $\rightleftharpoons$ World 2; and World 3 $\rightleftharpoons$ World 1 $\rightleftharpoons$ World 2. Transmission from World 3 to World 1 to World 2 occurs through processes of sensing, coded transmission to the brain, decoding there, and so on in accord with the information flow diagram of Fig. 6-3.

Central to the theme of the brain-mind liaison would be the ego or self (Fig. 6-2), which gives you the continuity in time, right from your earliest beginnings up to the present time. This is what gives you your unity as a person and it is that which in a religious sense could be called the soul. So in summary we can say that in *cognitive experience* there is outer sensing or perception via the receptor organs (Fig. 6-2), inner sensing which is all your memories, experiences of a more subtle kind, in fact all of the content of consciousness that is not dependent immediately upon what comes in your sense organs, and finally this central entity which is you as a person or self.

AN INVESTIGATION OF PERCEPTION

I will now give an example of perception in the visual system. In this chapter I will be traversing backwards and forwards between philosophical ideas and experimental investigations, the experiments linked with ideology, as should be the case in all science. In Fig. 6-4A there are the visual pathways with the transmission from eyes to the visual cortices of a human brain. Because of the *partial decussation*, the *left visual field* for both eyes projects to the *right visual cortex*, and vice versa for the right visual field (cf. Fig. 6-12). In the histological section of the visual areas of the cerebral cortex (Fig. 6-4B) each of those dots is a nerve cell, just as in Fig. 1-2A. There are about 300 million nerve cells in the human visual cortex, receiving the impulses transmitted along the pathways from one or the other eye. Microelectrodes can be used to record the impulses discharged from single nerve cells, as, for example, has been done with great success by Hubel and Wiesel.

I use one aspect of their work to illustrate the very subtle and well-controlled experiments that are being carried out in many laboratories. In Fig. 6-5A there is a single cell firing impulses, having been "found" by a microelectrode which has been inserted into the primary visual cortex of the cat. The track of insertion is shown for example in Fig. 6-5B as the sloping line with short transverse lines indicating the locations of

VENTRAL ASPECT OF HUMAN BRAIN   MAGNIFIED PORTION OF
WITH VISUAL PATHWAYS SHADED   HUMAN VISUAL CORTEX

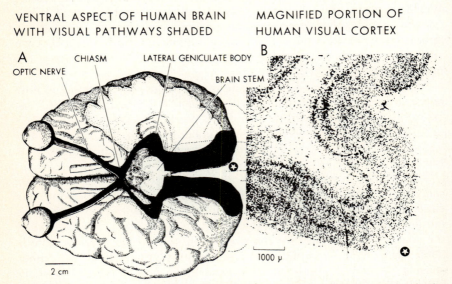

Figure 6-4   The visual pathways in man. Because of the partial decussation in the optic chiasma, the left visual field for both eyes projects to the right visual cortex and vice versa for the right visual field as illustrated in Fig. 6-12. The symbol of star inside circle indicates identical areas in *A* and *B*, but in *B* the magnification is about 20 times greater.

many nerve cells along that track. With the microelectrode you can record extracellularly the impulse discharges of a single cell if you position it carefully, as has been illustrated in Figs. 4-4, and 4-19, for example. The cell has a slow background discharge (upper trace of Fig. 6-5*A*), but if the retina is swept with a band of light, as illustrated in the diagram to the left, there is an intense discharge of that cell when light sweeps across a certain zone of the retina and there is immediate cessation of the discharge as the light band leaves the zone (lowest trace of Fig. 6-5*A*). If you rotate the direction of sweep, the cell discharges just a little as in the middle trace. Finally, if the sweep is at right angles to the most favorable direction, it has no effect whatever (uppermost trace). It is a sign, you see, that this particular cell is most sensitive for movements of the light strip in one orientation and is quite insensitive for movements at right angles thereto. As illustrated by the direction of the lines across the microelectrode track in Fig. 6-5*B*, all cells along that track have the same orientational sensitivity. This is found when the track runs along a column of cells that is orthogonal to the surface, as in the upper group of 12 cells. However, in Fig. 6-5*B* the track continued on across the central white matter and then proceeded to pass through three groups of cells with quite different orientation sensitivities. Evidently the track was crossing several columns with different orientational sensitivities in the way illustrated by the dotted sectors. This columnar arrangement for mutual reinforcement of similar receiving cells has already been illustrated (Figs. 4-5 and 4-6) and discussed in Chap. 4.

It has been demonstrated by Jung, Bishop, and others that retinal

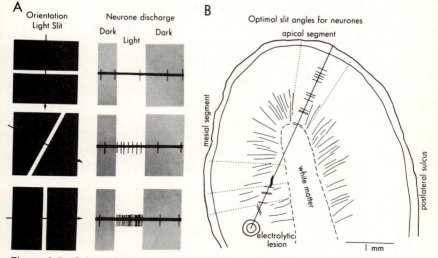

Figure 6-5 Orientational responses of neuron in visual cortex of cat. Full description in text. (*From Hubel and Wiesel, 1962.*)

zones adjacent to those giving excitation have an inhibitory action on the firing of a neuron such as that of Fig. 6-5A. For example, if the cell in Fig. 6-5A had a relatively high background discharge, this discharge would be depressed by illumination of adjacent areas of the retina. This can be explained by the diagram of Fig. 4-6 where excitation of one area of the cerebral cortex results in inhibition of adjacent areas, much as with basket-cell inhibition in the cerebellum in Fig. 4-13. This observation has great interest because it explains the so-called Mach bands of perceptual physiology. At the edge between fields of uniform bright and dull illumination there is perceived to be a narrow light-dark zone, the Mach band, which is explicable by this lateral inhibition.

The activation of cells in the primary visual cortex does not in itself give you a sensation. This is merely the first coded response of the visual cortex. Before you can experience a flash of light, there must be induced neuronal discharges in extremely complicated pathways after many successive levels of neuronal transmission. As shown by Hubel and Wiesel, each one of these cells with its simple orientational sensing (Fig. 6-5B), relays into interacting systems of cells which will respond specifically to angles of different degrees between the two light bands, and that also may be specified as to the length of the effective light bands. As you go further from the primary visual cortex out into the surrounding areas of the visual cortex, these more synthetic responses are observed for the so-called complex and hypercomplex cells. It is a further stage of the processing that goes on in the brain.

Figure 6-6 is a diagram of what I imagine is occurring at levels where there may be some kind of neural coding that gives you a conscious perception. It is assumed that the neuronal responses have been built up to a level of immense complexity, only a minute fragment being shown in the diagram. There is experimental evidence that the building of a requisite level of complexity for a perceptual experience may take as long as one-fifth of a second with vision, and Libet has shown that up to a half a second is necessary when there is a threshold electrical stimulation of a touch area in the brain in conscious human subjects.

In Fig. 6-6 nerve cells of the cerebral cortex are represented as circles, solid or open, that are arranged in clusters, each cluster corresponding to a column of the cerebral cortex, as has been illustrated in Fig. 4-6 and as indicated in Figs. 4-5 and 6-5. It was suggested in the discussion of Fig. 4-6 that the cells of a cluster are activated by self-reexciting chains, but also are subjected to inhibition from adjacent clusters, which is not shown in Fig. 6-6. An excited cluster projects on to other columns in the cerebral cortex by association fibers as symbolized by the arrows so that there is sequential activation of cluster to cluster, with in one case a return circuit giving a loop for sustained activation. Otherwise there is the progressive invasion of successive clusters. A particular sensory modality

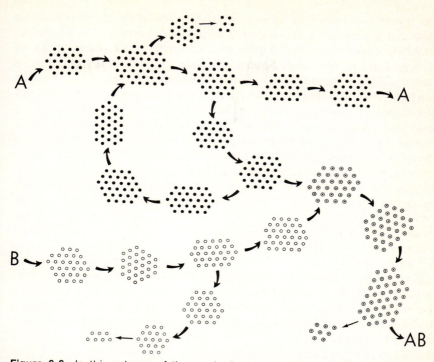

Figure 6-6 In this schema of the cerebral cortex looked at from above, the large pyramidal cells are represented as circles, solid or open, that are arranged in clusters, each cluster corresponding to a column as diagrammed in the cover picture and in Fig. 4-6, where only two large projecting pyramidal cells are shown of the hundreds that would be in the column. The large arrows symbolize impulse discharges along hundreds of lines in parallel, which are the mode of excitatory communication from column to column. Two inputs, A and B, and two outputs, A and AB are shown. Further description in text.

(*A*) is envisaged as activating the clusters with cells identified by solid circles, and input from another modality (*B*) activates clusters with open circles. Finally convergence of the transmission of the *A* and *B* modalities gives activation of clusters of cells with a modality reference corresponding to both *A* and *B* and so are shown with a symbolism (*AB*) corresponding to both—the dense core circles. For example, cells of *A* input may be responding to one sensory input, say a touch, and the cells of *B* to a visual input. In that case the confluence of *A* and *B* could represent the combined tactile and visual recognition of an object. It is to be noted that one cluster can project to two other clusters. However, in Fig. 6-6 there are three examples where excitation is inadequate for indefinite onward propagation from cluster to cluster. Thus in the diagram the two inputs *A* and *B* give only two outputs, *A* and *AB*.

The cross-sectional areas of cortical columns are probably no more than 0.2 mm², which would give a neuronal population of not more than 10,000, of which only a few hundred would be pyramidal cells projecting out of the column (cf. Fig. 4-6) to other cortical areas, for example, as envisaged in Fig. 6-6. Such estimates indicate that there may be no more than 1 million columns in the human cerebrum. However, it must be recognized that columns do not act in a strictly unitary manner. Rather their action can be considered as made up from the many hundreds of pyramidal cells projecting out of the column in a much more diverse manner than in Fig. 6-6, where the projection was to no more than two other colums, whereas it should be to 100 or more.

Figure 6-6 represents the kind of patterning of the activated cells that Sherrington was imagining when he said poetically (he was a poet) that the active brain is "an enchanted loom, weaving a dissolving pattern, always a meaningful pattern, though never an abiding one, a shifting harmony of subpatterns." And this, of course, cannot be drawn in two dimensions!

Each cell branches to go to perhaps 50 or more other cells and receives from a like number. If this connectivity is to be drawn in a strict geometrical diagram, it would have to be shown in an equivalent number of dimensions. Even if in 20 dimensions the patterned operation of the neuronal network of the brain is beyond any imagination; nevertheless it is possible to utilize n-dimensional geometry for estimating the numbers of neurons involved after a few synaptic relays. I want you to realize that even a simple flash of light must result in this immense patterned performance of cerebral neurons in space and time before there is the simplest conscious experience. Do not imagine that a conscious experience results from a few cells firing in some special area, with different cells specified for different experiences. For example, when some pontifical cells are somewhere discharging, you see a triangle. Sherrington stated that the brain has to work as a millionfold democracy to give you even the simplest experience, which is surely an understatement. Rather is the brain a 100-millionfold democracy even in giving a quite simple experience. Lashley also postulated that the neuronal patterns responsible for the recall of the simplest memory, the engram, involved tens of millions of nerve cells.

Experimental evidence for the immense influence of sensory inputs on the neuronal activity of the cerebral cortex is provided by the electroencephalogram (Fig. 6-7). As is well known, when there is a minimal input of sensory information and mental relaxation, rhythmic potentials of about 10 per second, the *alpha* (α) *rhythm*, can be led from the cerebral cortex, usually after conduction through the skull to the electrodes placed on the scalp. It is believed that this rhythm is basically due to immense numbers of cortical neurons firing more or less in phase

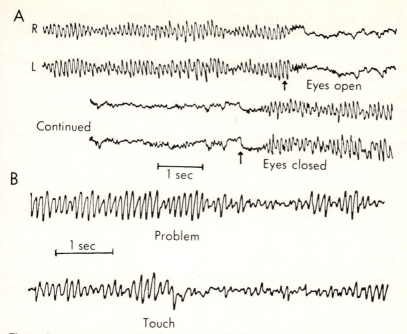

Figure 6-7 Electroencephalograms of man. *A.* Effect of opening eyes in suppressing the alpha rhythm recorded simultaneously from the right (R) and left(L) occipital poles of the human cerebrum, and return of rhythm on closing eyes. Note similarities of electroencephalogram on the two sides. [*H. H. Jasper, "Electroencephalography," in Chap. 14 in W. Penfield and T. C. Erickson (eds.), Epilepsy and Cerebral Localization, 1941.*] *B.* Effect of brain activity in mental arithmetic and with afferent stimulation in causing temporary cessation of alpha rhythm. [*E. D. Adrian and B. H. C. Matthews, Brain, 57:355 (1934).*]

as a result of thalamocortical circuits reverberating via pathways diagrammed in Fig. 3-13. Andersen and Andersson have fully developed this theme. In Fig. 6-7*A* the alpha rhythm is reversibly abolished by opening the eyes, which is explicable by the disturbing action of the tremendous inflow of impulses via the visual pathways. However, in Fig. 6-7*B*, the much milder afferent input by a touch on the skin greatly disturbs the alpha rhythm, which indicates that this input certainly would have spread to tens of millions of cortical neurons, as postulated above. The sequential spread from the primary receiving area in the primate cerebral cortex has been beautifully demonstrated by Jones and Powell with their techniques of cascade degeneration. For example, killing of the neurons of the somatic sensory transmitting area (cf. Fig. 4-1) results in degeneration of the nerve fibers projecting from that area to three other cortical areas. Killing of neurons of the major area for this primary projection results in degeneration of fibers in three other areas, the secondary projection areas, and so on for as many as three degeneration sequences. Of course separate monkeys were used for each sequence. It has thus been shown that the primary sensory area projects in an orderly manner to a multitude of circumscribed zones not only in the parietal lobe but also in the temporal, frontal, and limbic lobes. And at the third projection there is convergence of several modalities onto the same cortical area. This demonstration provides the anatomical substrate for cross-modal interaction, such as has been diagrammatically indicated in Fig. 6-6 for tactile and visual inputs. These anatomical findings are matched by physiological investigations on the somatosensory system by Mountcastle and by Hubel, Wiesel, Gross, and others on the visual system. In wide areas of the cortex neurons are found that respond to two or more modalities of input. The large disturbance of alpha rhythm in Fig. 6-7*B* also illustrates the enormous extent of the neuronal involvement in working out a problem in mental arithmetic.

It can be concluded that the nervous system is not working in some unitary and dictatorial manner. The time for neuronal transmission across the diagram of Fig. 6-6 would be only about one-tenth of a second if you allow one-hundredth of a second for the buildup of excitation in a cluster and the transfer from one cluster to the next. It is impossible to imagine what the weaving situation would be, given the power of multiplication which would occur for many clusters in parallel with incessant divergence and convergence of lines instead of the few shown in Fig. 6-6. Before the cerebral cortex is involved in the necessary complex patterned reaction to the sensory input so that it gives a conscious perception, there will be activity of this immense, unimaginable complexity. That is why I regard attempts at computer simulation as being beyond all hope. With the cerebellum, computer simulation in principle should not be an impossible goal. More is needed in the way of raw data, but we have seen in Chap. 4 that this is being rapidly accumulated, and the neuronal pathways are well known. By contrast the cerebrum presents problems of a different order altogether. It will be necessary to venture into what Sperry calls holistic or global concepts. Furthermore it will be necessary to develop new forms of mathematics, as yet unimagined, in order to cope with such immense patterned complexities.

THE CEREBRUM AND SPEECH

In the left cerebral hemisphere (Fig. 6-8) are the speech centers. These areas have been defined by studies of clinical lesions that started over 100 years ago. Firstly, Broca observed that a lesion in the *inferior frontal convolution* resulted in a failure to speak, though language was still understood, the so-called *motor aphasia*. The most important discovery

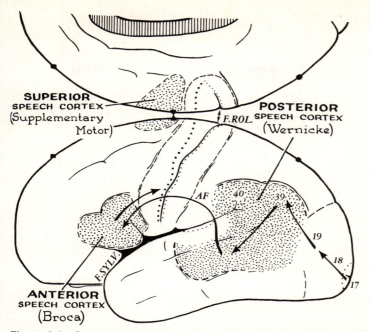

Figure 6-8 Cortical speech areas of dominant hemisphere. Note that view is of left hemisphere from both lateral and medial aspects. F. Rol. is the fissure of Rolando and F. Sylv. is the fissure of Sylvius. (*From Penfield and Roberts, 1959.*)

was made a little later by Wernicke who found that, with lesions of the *superior temporal convolution, the posterior speech area of Wernicke*, there was a failure to understand language—heard or written—though confused "jargon" speaking was still possible. It is amazing to find in the subsequent clinical literature that a study of randomly located lesions in patients led to such a remarkable understanding and mapping of the language areas of the brain. This study went on concurrently with the localization of the motor and the primary sensory areas that are displayed in Fig. 4-1. Right from the beginning it was realized that the speech areas were in one hemisphere only, almost always the left. A thorough scientific investigation of the speech centers led Penfield and Roberts to estimate that only in about 2 percent are the speech centers in the right hemisphere. This extreme preponderance of the left hemisphere has nothing, as a rule, to do with handedness. Most left-handed subjects have speech in the left hemisphere.

Electrical stimulation provides a valuable method in testing for speech areas. Stimulation of the right hemisphere can give vocalization. Calls and cries, but not expressive language, are produced by stimulation of the motor areas concerned in voice control, as indicated in Fig. 6-9. But

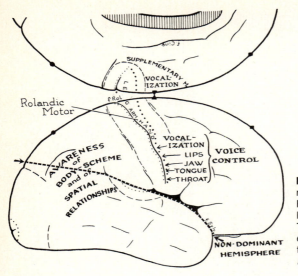

Figure 6-9 Vocalization of minor hemisphere. As with Fig. 6-8, the view is both of lateral and medial aspects. The various effects were evoked by electrical stimulation. (*From Penfield and Roberts, 1959.*)

nowhere in that hemisphere do you get speech disorders from stimulation. On the contrary, gentle electrical stimulation of the speech areas of the left hemisphere in the conscious subject either silences or greatly disturbs speech in progress, there being, for example, word repetition or confusion of expression during the stimulation.

This very clear distinction for such an important cerebral function as speech prompts the question: Is there any anatomically recognizable structure to match this unilaterality of speech? Until recently the answer would have been: No, the two hemispheres look alike despite their differences in functional performance, i.e., speech is not related to macrostructure. But recently Geschwind and Wada have shown that there is usually a remarkable asymmetry if you open up the fissurae and so see what was concealed from superficial examination. For example, the surface of the superior temporal convolution can be displayed by removing the frontal and parietal lobes, i.e., by cutting off all of the brain above the broken line in Fig. 6-9. Figure 6-10 shows that when that is done a remarkable asymmetry is displayed, TP and OP being the temporal and occipital poles respectively. The shaded area (PT) would be central in the posterior speech area of Wernicke, and the corresponding area (PT) on the right side is much smaller. In most cases there is this clear asymmetry in the human brain with the *dominant* or *speech hemisphere* showing an enlargement here in the speech area that is not matched on the other side.

Unfortunately, as usual in biology, the story is not so simple. The asymmetrical enlargement in the regions of speech center only occurs in about 65 percent of left cerebral hemispheres, not in the 98 percent that

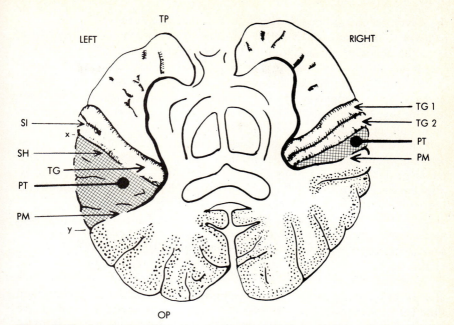

Figure 6-10 Asymmetry of human superior temporal lobe. Upper surfaces of human temporal lobes exposed by a cut on each side as illustrated by the broken lines in Figs. 6-8 and 6-9. Typical left-right differences are shown. The posterior margin (PM) of the planum temporale (PT) slopes backward more sharply on the left than on the right, so that end y of the left Sylvian fissure lies posterior to the corresponding point on the right. The anterior margin of the sulcus of Heschl (SH) slopes forward more sharply on the left. In this brain there is a single traverse gyrus of Heschl (TG) on the left and two on the right (TG 1, TG 2). TP, temporal pole; OP, occipital pole; SI, sulcus intermedius of Beck. (*From Geschwind and Levitsky, 1968.*)

would be expected from the left lateralization of speech. A possible explanation of this discrepancy will be given later when discussing Sperry's split-brain investigations. After more than a century of intensive anatomical study on the human brain, it is most surprising to be confronted with the discovery of this hemispheral asymmetry. No such asymmetry has been detected with nonhuman primates, which matches their linguistic deficiency.

Wada has made the remarkable discovery that human infants are born with this asymmetry. It has already been grown by genetic instructions in anticipation of its eventual usage in speech, and can be detected even in a 7-month-old fetus. We can surmise that the speech areas of the cortex are developed with a neuronal structure specialized for the unique operations of coding and decoding required for linguistic performance. Since in the fetus this structure is developed almost always on the left side, it is not surprising that the left hemisphere is still as a rule utilized for the development of speech despite severe damage at birth. Nevertheless transfer to the undamaged right hemisphere has been reported, and there are even accounts of bilaterality of speech representation.

It would be expected that highly specialized patterns of neuronal connectivity would be developed in the speech areas, but as yet I do not know of any attempt to carry out histological studies at the required level of subtlety, particularly with electron microscopy. The speech areas in their full performance—speaking, hearing, writing, reading—must be carrying out a most incredible decoding and coding operation, far beyond our imagination. For example, in reading aloud, black marks on white paper are projected from the retina to the brain in the form of coding by impulse discharge frequencies in optic nerve fibers and so eventually to the neurons of the primary visual cortex as in Figs. 6-4 and 6-5. The next stage is the transmission of the coded visual information to the visual association areas (18 and 19 in Fig. 6-8) where there is a further stage of reconstitution of the visual image. Neurons there specifically respond to simple geometrical forms, the so-called feature-recognition neurons. However, at the next stage, lesions of the posterior part of Wernicke's area (area 39 in Fig. 6-8) result in dyslexia, suggesting that the relay from the visual-association neurons provides information that is converted into word patterns and that these in turn are interpreted as meaningful sentences in the process of conscious recognition. It is our thesis that this occurs because the self-conscious mind is able to interact with modules in this cortical area. Lesions result in Wernicke's aphasia. The further stage in the process of reading aloud is via the arcuate fasciculus (AF in Fig. 6-8) to the motor speech area (Broca's area). Lesions of the arcuate fasciculus result in conduction aphasia. There is comprehension of spoken language but a gross defect in its repetition and in normal speaking. At the terminal stage appropriate patterns of neural activity in Broca's area lead to the motor areas for vocalization and so to the coordinated contractions of the speech muscles. Thus eventually out comes spoken language which another person can understand. This necessitates another process of coding and decoding in the speech areas of the recipient with eventually transmission from spatiotemporal neuronal patterns (Fig. 6-6) in the liaison brain (Fig. 6-3) that is in communication with World 2. The performance of speech areas is uniquely concerned in these neuronal operations, and we would expect that it could be a performance of a kind that we cannot match elsewhere in the brain. That is a remarkable claim. Electrophysiologically no observations have been made at a meaningful level. It is an open field.

It is often said that all the good scientific questions have been answered. You can now see that for the brain at least this is not at all true. I think that all the best scientific questions are still waiting. In the attempts made in this book to understand the brain, we have seen repeatedly that most interesting and important questions are now being intensively studied, but they are not yet solved. And when solutions are discovered, many more new questions will arise.

THE DOMINANT AND THE MINOR CEREBRAL HEMISPHERES

In Fig. 6-11 the *corpus callosum* in a monkey's brain is drawn after it has been severed. The brain is rather like a human brain, only smaller. This great tract, the corpus callosum, links together almost all areas of the left and the right hemispheres. A few areas, such as the primary visual area and the hand and foot somesthetic areas are "blind" to the corpus callosum. For all other areas there is a mirror-image linkage, such as is indicated in Fig. 6-11. There are about 200 million callosal fibers in the human brain and in these fibers there is an incessant traffic. If we suppose that each fiber has an average firing frequency of 20 impulses a second, your corpus callosum would be carrying 4 billion impulses a second right now! This immense traffic keeps the two hemispheres of the brain working together. Of course all the various areas of one or the other hemisphere are also linked by great tracts. Nevertheless the immense linkage by the corpus callosum connects the two hemispheres perhaps as effectively as are the diverse areas within one hemisphere.

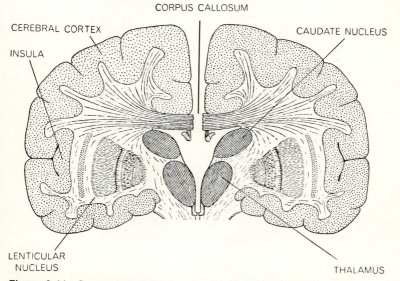

Figure 6-11   Separation of the two cerebral hemispheres produced by section of the corpus callosum in the monkey's brain.

As against all other intracerebral tracts, the corpus callosum offers a remarkable attraction for experimental investigation. It alone can be cleanly and completely severed without damaging any other structures (cf. Figs. 6-11 and 6-12). This operation has been carried out in more than 20 human subjects who were suffering from almost incessant epileptic seizures that could not be controlled, even by heavy medication. It was surmised that seizures developed in one cerebral hemisphere and then excited the other via the corpus callosum so that the seizure rapidly

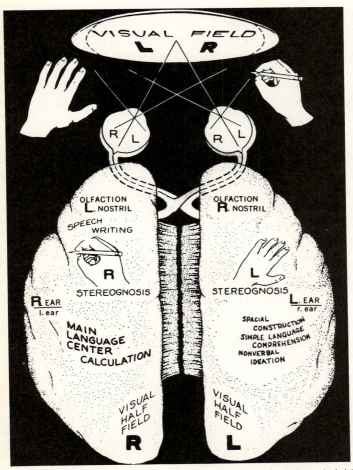

Figure 6-12 Schema showing the way in which the left and right visual fields are projected onto the right and left visual cortices, respectively, due to the partial decussation in the optic chiasma. The schema also shows other sensory inputs from right limbs to the left hemisphere and that from left limbs to the right hemisphere. Similarly, hearing is largely crossed in its input, but olfaction is ipsilateral. (*From Sperry, 1970a.*)

became generalized. Hence, it was proposed that section of the corpus callosum would at least keep one hemisphere free from the seizures. It turns out that the operation does better than predicted. There is a remarkable diminution of seizures in both hemispheres. Apparently there is a reciprocal incitement of each hemisphere by the other.

Sperry and his associates were well equipped to study the human subjects with refined techniques because they had spent several years investigating monkeys subjected to a similar operation. Some early investigators on human brains had come up with so little result from cutting the corpus callosum that it was rather facetiously suggested that the only function of the corpus callosum was to keep the two hemispheres from falling apart! Sperry's study has avoided several technical deficiencies in this earlier work and over the last 10 years has given incredibly interesting results. There have been discoveries beyond anything that could have been predicted. Figure 6-12 is a diagram in which Sperry summarizes some of the experimental findings. I will refer to these later. For present purposes the diagram is important in showing that, because of the partial decussation in the optic chiasma, the right visual field for both eyes projects to the visual cortex in the left hemisphere: note the letter R in the left visual cortex, and similarly for the left visual field and the right visual cortex (letter L).

Figure 6-13 illustrates the method of testing subjects designed by Sperry. The subject fixes his gaze on the central spot on the screen, and on the left or right side of this screen can be flashed for one-tenth of a

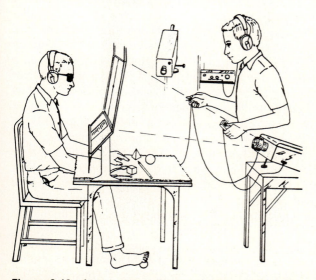

Figure 6-13 Arrangement of general testing unit in demonstrating symptoms produced by commissural section. (*From Sperry, 1970a.*)

second some signal to him. You can also talk to him and give instructions by demonstration. There may just have been on the left visual field of the screen, for example, the word NUT (Fig. 6-14) and this split-brain subject can put out his left hand and unerringly retrieve the nut from all the other objects. This experimental arrangement is very well designed for testing the two sides of the brain, each one independently of the other. This can be done because, if you project some message—word or picture—onto the left visual field it will be transmitted entirely to the right visual cortex, as indicated in Fig. 6-12, and from there it is transmitted widely to the right hemisphere. Similarly everything in the right field goes to the left visual cortex and the left hemisphere, which is the speech hemisphere in all the subjects Sperry has investigated. It is also important to recall that because of the decussation of the pyramidal tract (Fig. 4-2) the right hemisphere programs the movements of the left hand. However, there is a small uncrossed component, and thus in some subjects the left hemisphere can to a small extent bring about movements on the left side.

Let us now return to Fig. 6-14 in which the word NUT was flashed on the left visual field and so appeared in the right visual cortex, and thence via various recognition pathways to the right motor cortex, which can program the left hand (cf. Fig. 6-12) so that it seeks amongst the array of objects and finds the nut. Throughout all this procedure the left hand is screened from view. But now the interesting thing is that the subject, when questioned, knows nothing about what is going on. The signal onto the left visual field was not seen, nor is there any recognition of what the left hand is seeking or finding. He either admits ignorance or makes a random guess as indicated by the question mark. This is a remarkable result. The right hemisphere displays apparently intelligent actions, the reading of a word, the recognition of the object signified by the word as indicated by the searching for and discovery of that object, and even a display of its correct usage by the left hand (threading it on a bolt), and yet the speaking subject is completely ignorant of the whole operation. It has to be recognized that, in addition to the pyramidal tract decussation, there is also a decussation of sensory pathways from a limb (cf. Fig. 3-13), so that the sensory input from the left hand, for example, is received, after decussation, also by the right hemisphere. Thus the left hemisphere receives no information about what the left hand is doing or feeling. Everything is fed back into the right hemisphere, which is the hemisphere that received the original visual signal, and it is this hemisphere alone that is programming the searching and finding. In this kind of experiment it is essential to use a flashed signal for no more than one-tenth of a second. With longer visual displays the subject will have moved his eyes so that the signal is also projected to the right visual field. Such cross-cueing defeats the experiment. All Sperry's experiments are so designed. This

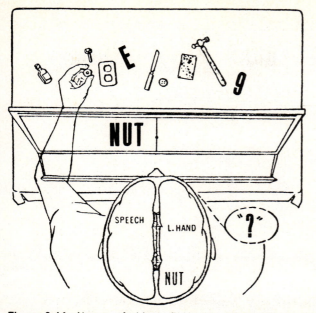

Figure 6-14 Names of objects flashed to left half-field can be read and understood but not spoken. Subject can retrieve the named object by touch with the left hand, but cannot afterwards name the item or retrieve it with the right hand. (*From Sperry, 1970a.*)

essential precaution had not been rigorously applied by previous investigators.

I want to build up the idea that Sperry has developed from the whole range of his experiments, namely, that all "goings-on" in the right hemisphere (the so-called *minor hemisphere*) are unknown to the speaking subject who is only in liaison with the "goings-on" in the left hemisphere, the *dominant hemisphere*. The dominant hemisphere alone can communicate with language. As Sperry states, it is the talking hemisphere; and we have seen that the speech centers are in this hemisphere (Fig. 6-8). Furthermore in liaison with this hemisphere is the conscious being or self that is recognizably the same person as before the operation. Originally this self had a brain with two hemispheres, but now it has only one. This is what the section of the corpus callosum has done, yet the subject gets on very well in the ordinary affairs of life.

Figure 6-15 gives an example of how complete is the cleavage between the events in the two hemispheres. The flash display is HAT BAND so that HAT goes as shown to the right hemisphere and BAND to the left (speaking) hemisphere. When you ask the subject what word did he see, he will say "band." Tests make it quite clear that the speaking

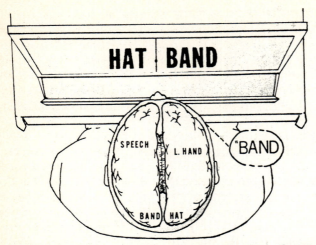

Figure 6-15 Only the name flashed to the right visual field is read and reported verbally by the subject. The name in the left visual field is not consciously seen nor is it even subconsciously associated with the name seen in the right visual field. (*From Sperry, 1970a.*)

subject had no idea that the right hemisphere had received the word "hat" at the same time. If you ask: What kind of band? all manner of guesses are expressed verbally such as "rock 'n' roll band," "rubber band," "robber band," or something like that and only by chance "hat band." Similar tests have been carried out with many word combinations—"key case," "he art"—that are split between the left and right visual fields, always with the same results. There is never a trace of cross transfer from the right to the left hemisphere, and so to the conscious experience of the subject.

Figure 6-16 illustrates an even more remarkable investigation that shows a minor linguistic performance for the right hemisphere despite its inability to speak. It has certainly some ideational existence of its own, and is quite clever in some ways. You saw that it correctly recognized the meaning of the word NUT in Fig. 6-14. In Fig. 6-16 it exhibits a remarkable writing performance. Initially there is a display (not flashed) of a list of names of common objects that is fed into both hemispheres: knife, glass, cup, spoon, book, pen, etc.; then the subject is instructed with the left hand to write a word selected from this list and flashed on the left visual field. In Fig. 6-16 the right hemisphere seeing BOOK flashed on the left visual field will cause the left hand to write "book" correctly, but in a different script from the image fed into it. That is a remarkably good bit of writing for the left hand that is of course screened from view. Usually it breaks down after writing two letters. When you ask the speaking subject, "what did the left hand write?" you discover that he knows that something has been written because he feels the writing movement coming through the body. However, he has no detailed information and says "cup," which is a pure guess from the initial test list. Purely on chance scoring will he tell correctly what the left was doing. So there's no communication from the minor to the dominant (left) hemisphere. This remarkable experiment shows you how important the corpus callosum is in conveying precise information from one hemisphere to the other.

However there is some transfer at a crude emotional or behavioristic level. A picture is flashed onto the left visual field that would be expected to give the subject fear or embarrassment. A vague emotional response is experienced by the subject who is unable to understand its causation. For example, a nude female picture, perhaps from *Playboy*, was flashed onto the left visual field and of course not seen by the conscious subject. Nevertheless she gave embarrassed smiles and tittered a bit but didn't know why she had these strange emotional feelings welling up. Presumably the emotional reaction of the minor hemisphere had gone down into the limbic system and the hypothalamus and from there had come up again to the left hemisphere. It has to be remembered that in the hypothalamic region, and indeed in the whole brainstem there is the

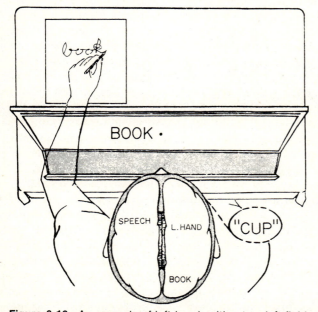

Figure 6-16 An example of left-hand writing to a left-field presentation, followed by incorrect verbalization. [*R. D. Nebes and R. W. Sperry, Neuropsychologia, 9:247 (1971).*]

normal communication across the midline. The operative splitting is restricted to the cerebral commissures. But there is really no information content in the transfer at these lower levels, only a mood change. This same vague transfer with negligible information content can also occur with fear or other emotional disturbances. Such a mood change can develop slowly and last for quite a long time, as if it is dependent on some hormonal mechanism. The role of biogenic amines and the limbic system in mood is beyond the scope of this chapter, but a reference is given to a review by Kety that covers admirably the whole of this important field of brain states.

Despite the good performance of the right hemisphere in respect to names of common objects, even simple verbs are very little, if at all, comprehended by it. If you present to the left visual field such verbal commands as nod, wink, shake head, smile, you practically never get a response, which is in contrast to names. And the comprehension of the right hemisphere extends beyond names of common objects. Descriptive phrases can be recognized as signals to retrieve objects from an assortment provided. For example, "for lighting fire" results in retrieval of a match; "for holding liquid," a glass; "measuring instrument," a ruler, Again, if you present to the left visual field a picture of a large wall clock, the left hand will search for the best available object and, for example, come up with a toy wristwatch; or if a dollar sign is flashed, there is retrieval of a coin, a quarter, for example. So we must recognize that the right hemisphere not only comprehends names of common objects but also the associations of those objects. I think you will agree that it is a very clever hemisphere. A further remarkable performance is exhibited by the delayed responses. For example, a signal can be flashed to the left visual field and even after an enforced delay of 5 min after the flash, the left hand can go to a grab bag of 20 objects and retrieve the correct object. Sperry says that no nonhuman primate can match the performance of the right hemisphere both in respect of cross-modality recognition and of delayed performance as here described.

We can now return to Fig. 6-12 which is a diagram drawn by Sperry several years ago. However it is still valuable as a basis of discussion of the whole split-brain story. We have already used it in reference to the right and left visual fields and their highly selective projection to the crossed visual cortices, as indicated by the letters R and L. Also shown in the diagram is the strictly unilateral projection of smell and the predominantly crossed projection of hearing. The crossed representations of both motor and sensory innervation of the hands are indicated, and also the further finding that arithmetical calculation is predominant in the left hemisphere. Only very simple addition sums can be carried out by the right hemisphere. Recent conceptual developments with respect to hemispheral function will be discussed later in reference to Fig. 6-17.

All of this fine work with flash testing has been superseded by a new technique developed by Zaidel and Sperry in which a contact lens is placed in the right eye with an attached optical device that limits the input into that eye to the left visual field no matter how the eye is moved. At the same time, an eye shield covers the left eye. In this way there can be up to 2 h of continuous investigation of the subject, which gives opportunity for more sophisticated testing procedures than with the flash technique. The tests have been concerned with the ability of the right (minor) hemisphere in understanding complex visual imagery, as shown by appropriate reactions with the left hand.

For example, strip cartoons made up of four to six picture cards randomly arranged can be sorted by the left hand and arranged in correct sequence despite the fact that the conscious subject verbally reports that he has no idea either of what is being presented in the left visual field or of the reactions of the left hand thereto. It must be recognized that with the screening of the left eye and the optical device on the contact lens of the right eye, there is elimination of all input to the subject from the right visual field, i.e., the subject is quite blind so far as any conscious visual experiences are concerned.

Despite an intelligent performance with pictorial and verbal presentation to the minor hemisphere, this hemisphere is completely unable to complete sentences, even the simplest, when tested in the manner illustrated by the verbal arrangement given below.

Mother loves_____
nail   baby   broom   stone

The subject points with the left hand as the sentence is read: "Mother loves_____" and then sequentially to the four words below for identification. The subject then tries to complete the sentence using the left hand to point to one of the four words below, and only at random chance chooses "baby." The evidence from language testing of chimpanzees indicates likewise that they are unable to complete sentences, though some dubious claims have been made. This inability of course arises from the fact that neither the minor hemisphere nor the chimpanzee brain has a Wernicke area that provides the necessary semantic ability.

In conclusion we can say that the right hemisphere is a very highly developed brain except that it cannot express itself in language; it is not able to disclose any experience of consciousness that we can recognize. Sperry postulates that there is another consciousness in the right hemisphere, but that its existence is obscured by its lack of expressive language. On the other hand, the left hemisphere has a normal linguistic performance so it can be recognized as being associated with the prior existence of the ego or the self with all the memories of the past before the commissural section. On this view there has been split off from the talking self a nontalking self which can't communicate by language, so it is there but mute, or aphasic.

We will return later to consider further the unique performances of the minor or right hemisphere. For the present we can say that we do not know if there is some inexpressible consciousness in the isolated right hemisphere, just as we do not know of any consciousness animals might have. I do not deny them consciousness. I just say that we have to be agnostic about it. We cannot discover it in any way, but we have to realize the limitations of our testing procedures both for animals and for the isolated right hemisphere.

BRAIN-MIND LIAISON

It is my thesis that the philosophical problem of brain and mind has been transformed by these investigations of the functions of the separated dominant and minor hemispheres in the split-brain subjects. Several years ago I suggested that, *even before the splitting*, the conscious self was in liaison only with the dominant hemisphere. The minor hemisphere is always an unconscious hemisphere per se, but it achieves in the ordinary situations, of course, consciousness by communication with the dominant hemisphere by means of the massive impulse traffic through the corpus callosum. This hypothesis can be made quite specific in the diagrammatic illustration of the brain and its communications in Fig. 6-17, which can be seen as a development from Fig. 6-3 with likewise the representation of Worlds 1, 2, and 3. The conscious self (World 2) is shown to be in liaison only with *specific linguistic and ideational zones* of the dominant hemisphere. Only the World 3 of the memory stores in the brain is shown.

I now feel that this may be too radical an inference from the observations on commissurotomy patients. With the corpus callosum intact, neuronal activities of a special character may be generated in the minor hemisphere that give it some liaison with the self-conscious mind, as indicated by the broken lines from World 2 in Fig. 6-17.

In Fig. 6-17 the corpus callosum is shown as an extremely strong communication system so that all happenings in the minor hemisphere can very quickly and effectively be transmitted to the liaison brain of the dominant hemisphere, and so to the conscious self. This occurs for the contribution of the minor hemisphere for all perceptions, all experiences, and all memories, and in fact for the whole content of World 2 (cf. Figs. 6-1 and 6-2). When the corpus callosum is severed, there is revealed what was there all the time, namely that the minor hemisphere is always per se an unconscious part of the brain and that linkage through the corpus callosum is necessary for it to receive from and give information to the conscious self.

When I postulated many years ago, following Sherrington, that there was a special area of the brain in liaison with consciousness, I certainly did not imagine that any definitive experimental test could be applied in a few years. But now we have this distinction between the dominant hemisphere in liaison with the conscious self, and the minor hemisphere

MODES OF INTERACTION BETWEEN HEMISPHERES

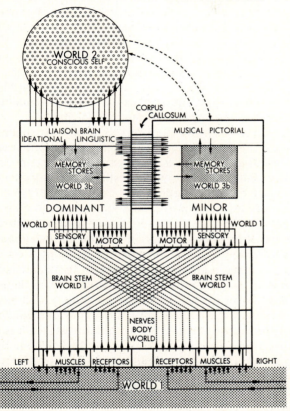

Figure 6-17 Communications to and from the brain and within the brain. Diagram to show the principal lines of communication from peripheral receptors to the sensory cortices and so to the cerebral hemispheres. Similarly, the diagram shows the output from the cerebral hemispheres via the motor cortex and so to muscles. Both these systems of pathways are largely crossed as illustrated, but minor uncrossed pathways are also shown. The dominant left hemisphere and minor right hemisphere are labeled, together with some of the properties of these hemispheres that are found displayed in Fig. 6-18. The corpus callosum is shown as a powerful cross-linking of the two hemispheres, and, in addition, the diagram displays the modes of interaction between Worlds 1, 2, and 3, as described in the text and also illustrated in Fig. 6-3. The dotted arrows to and from the minor hemisphere indicate possible lines of communication from the conscious self when the corpus callosum is intact (see text).

with no such liaison. It is this empirical discovery that I try to illustrate in Fig. 6-17. In it are shown the communication lines going both ways: out to the muscles via the motor pathways as illustrated in Figs. 4-1 and 4-2, and receiving from the world—the receptors to the sensory cortical areas—as partly illustrated in Figs. 3-13, 3-14, 6-4, and 6-5. Figure 6-17 also shows that, in addition to the usual crossed representation for input and output, there is a smaller ipsilateral representation, as has been evident in some of Sperry's investigations. It will also be recognized that, in its communication to World 2, the minor hemisphere normally suffers no material disability relative to the dominant hemisphere from its necessity to transmit through the corpus callosum to the liaison area of the dominant hemisphere. First, the corpus callosum is such an immense tract that in transmission through it the minor hemisphere would have no traffic problem. Second, as seen in Fig. 6-17, the greater part of the dominant hemisphere presumably has also to transmit to the liaison area.

So far the account of the performance of the minor hemisphere would suggest that it was grossly deficient in comparison with the dominant hemisphere. Recent developments by Sperry and Levy and in other laboratories do much to add many interesting and important functions to the repertoire of the minor hemisphere. Already in Fig. 6-12 there were displayed some interesting properties: spatial construction, nonverbal ideation. The tabular display in Fig. 6-18 gives a more expanded and significant list of functions for both the minor and dominant hemispheres. It is derived largely from recent investigations of Sperry and Levy, but there are some additions. In general, the dominant hemisphere is specialized in respect to fine imaginative details in all descriptions and reactions, i.e., it is analytic and sequential. Also it can add and subtract and multiply and carry out other computer-like operations. But of course its dominance derives from its verbal and ideational abilities and its liaison to consciousness (World 2). Because of its deficiencies in these respects the minor hemisphere deserves its title, but in many important properties it is preeminent, particularly in respect of its spatial abilities with a strongly developed pictorial and pattern sense. For example, the minor hemisphere programming the left hand is greatly superior in all kinds of geometrical and perspective drawings. This superiority is also evidenced by the ability to assemble colored blocks so as to match a mosaic picture. The dominant hemisphere is unable to carry out even simple tasks of this kind and is almost illiterate in respect to pictorial and pattern sense, at least as displayed by its copying disability. It is an arithmetical hemisphere but not a geometrical hemisphere. It is quite surprising how sharply these distinctions can be made. It could never have been predicted.

In general, Fig. 6-18 shows that in their properties the two hemispheres are complementary. The minor is coherent and the dominant is detailed. Furthermore, not only is the minor hemisphere pictorial, but there is evidence that it is musical. Music is essentially coherent and synthetic, being dependent on a sequential input of sounds. A coherent, synthetic, sequential imagery is made for us in some holistic manner by our musical sense. Furthermore there is accumulating evidence by Brenda Milner that excision of the right temporal lobe does, in fact, seriously limit musical ability, as displayed in the Seashore tests.

It is an attractive hypothesis of Sperry and Levy that the two hemispheres have complementary functions, which is an efficient arrangement because each can independently exercise its own peculiar abilities in developing and fashioning the neural input. Then in the ideational, linguistic, and liaison areas the two complementary performances can be combined and integrated. So in this way you, as a World 2 self, can have the advantage of presiding over the whole of your cerebral performance and receiving the cumulative and integrated result from your liaison brain.

FREE WILL

Now I come to a brief consideration of free will. I am not going to indulge in a philosophical argument on this too-much-discussed theme. All I have to say is that free will is a fact of experience. It is something each of us experiences. No one would have imagined free will to exist if he or she had not experienced it, by which I mean the ability to carry out actions that have been planned in thought, or at least to attempt to carry them out. Free will is often denied on the grounds that you cannot explain it, that it involves happenings inexplicable by present-day physics and physiology. To that I reply that our inability may stem from the fact that physics and

DOMINANT HEMISPHERE	MINOR HEMISPHERE
Liaison to consciousness	No such Liaison
Verbal	Almost non-verbal
Linguistic description	Musical
Ideational Conceptual similarities	Pictoral and Pattern sense Visual similarities
Analysis over time	Synthesis over time
Analysis of detail	Holistic — Images
Arithmetical and computer-like	Geometrics and Spatial

Figure 6-18 Various specific performances of the dominant and minor hemispheres as suggested by the new conceptual developments of Levy-Agresti and Sperry (1968) and Levy (1974). There are some additions to their original list.

physiology are still not adequately developed in respect of the immense patterned complexity of neuronal operation (cf. Fig. 6-6). The subtlety, the immense complexity of the patterns written in space and time by this "enchanted loom" of Sherrington, and the emergent properties of this system are beyond any levels of investigations by physics or physiology at the present time—as I have argued in my book *Facing Reality*—and perhaps for a long time to come. I would postulate that in the liaison areas these neuronal patterns are the receiving stations for the on-going operations in the consciousness of World 2, which is our world of primary reality as described at the outset of this chapter.

Even after this most perplexing stage of transmission from World 2 to the liaison brain, we still have to consider the further neuronal pathway thence to the motor cortex. We are now linking with the discussion on voluntary movement in Chap. 4, and particularly with the interpretation of the "readiness potential" illustrated in Fig. 4-3. Movements on the right side would result from some complex patterns of neuronal action, first in the liaison areas and then through unknown pathways to the motor cortex, the whole procedure occupying as long as 0.8 s as defined by the average duration of the readiness potential. The situation is similar for movements on the left side except that there is in addition the crossing to the minor hemisphere via the corpus callosum. Since the calculated time for such a crossing is no more than 0.01 s, motor actions voluntarily carried out by the minor hemisphere involve no more than a negligible temporal penalty. Again it must be recognized that in the ordinary performance of voluntary movements both the minor and dominant hemispheres are involved, and doubtless there is much to and fro communication across the corpus callosum during the readiness potential, which in its initial stages is bilateral even during the programming of a strictly unilateral action such as the flexion of one finger.

SUMMARY ON BRAIN-MIND LIAISON

Just because World 2 is drawn located above the brain in Fig. 6-17 (or Fig. 6-3), I do not wish to imply that World 2 is floating above the brain and has an autonomous existence and performance independent of the liaison area of the brain. On the contrary it is, so far as we can discover, tightly linked with neuronal activity there. If that stops, unconsciousness supervenes. As shown by the arrows in both directions in Fig. 6-17, there is an incessant interplay in the interaction between World 2 and the liaison brain, but we know nothing about its nature. This interaction is a tremendous challenge for the future. In this respect we can think of the whole range of psychiatry with such problems as those of the unconscious self, of sleep and dreams, of obsession. Despite our present ignorance of the precise neurological basis of all these problems of the psyche, we can have hope for some clearer understanding because it is now possible to define the liaison areas of the brain, and postulate that only in certain areas and in certain states of the brain does this relationship occur. This insight, limited as it is, provides hope for more understanding in this most fundamental problem.

The empirical support given to the concept of the liaison brain must discomfort the philosophers who like to be holistic about the brain-mind problem, as is for example proposed in the psychoneural identity hypothesis by Feigl. In that hypothesis it is postulated that all neuronal activity in the cerebrum comes through to consciousness somehow or other and is all expressed there. An often-used analogy is that neuronal activity and conscious states represent two different views of the same thing, one as seen by an external observer, the other as an inner experience by the "owner" of the brain. This proposed identification at least in its present form is refuted by the discovery that after commissurotomy none of the neuronal events in the minor hemisphere is recognized by the conscious subject.

As a final summary of the brain-mind problem, let us return to Fig. 6-17. We see here the largely crossed input from receptors, from visual fields and limbs in particular. Input into the minor hemisphere from the left side is fully processed in that hemisphere, but has to cross via the corpus callosum for integration with information from the right side and for conscious recognition. Figure 6-17 should serve as a reminder that there is also an immense impulse traffic through the corpus callosum from the dominant to the minor hemisphere. In this way inputs to the dominant hemisphere from its various lines of communication can, after due processing, be switched into the minor hemisphere for the exercise of its special functions as outlined in Fig. 6-18. However, it must be understood that Fig. 6-17 is an extremely simplified diagram. No attempt is made to illustrate the levels of complexity in the interaction of the two hemispheres by means of the immense callosal traffic or, even more so, in the interactions between the liaison areas and World 2.

BRAIN EVOLUTION, CULTURAL EVOLUTION, AND CONSCIOUSNESS

We will now return to the diagrams of the three worlds (Figs. 6-1 and 6-3), in which we have seen that World 3 is uniquely human. This is the question I ask: How did man come to be what he is? What is the evolutionary story behind man? Let's face it, man is unique. We must not accept the idea that man is *just* a superior animal. This is certainly not true. In his intellectual, rational, ethical, and aesthetic activities man has outgrown his animal ancestry to an amazing degree, though his emotions and behavior patterns still betray his ancestry, as has been emphasized by Konrad Lorenz. The uniqueness of man is attributable to World 3, which of course was made by man. When man, say a million years ago, was just a poor hominid battering pebbles, you would never have predicted he would have progressed beyond that, particularly if you as a privileged observer could have seen that for hundreds of thousands of years he would hardly improve his pebble battering! You can see the record in museums. Nevertheless, slowly he did improve, and, eventually, with progressive acceleration.

It is generally believed—by Dobzhansky and Popper, for example—that language played a key role. Man had undoubtedly developed considerable linguistic means of communication more than 100 millennia ago, and this meant he now became a community performer able to communicate experiences. Eventually he achieved self-consciousness by this communication with his fellows. I would put the dawn of self-consciousness, the sure knowledge of World 2, as at least 100,000 years ago because the earliest known Neanderthal ceremonial graves were at that time. Neanderthal men buried the dead with antlers around them, and with food and weapons and so on. We can surmise that at that time a primitive man would be looking at others dying and thinking, "He's like me, this can happen to me. I too can cease to live." And then began that transmutation from being merely knowing creatures to creatures that *know* that they know, which is the essence of self-consciousness. We can surmise that that came only when linguistic development was far advanced.

This advanced language would be used for description and discussion and argument. These linguistic usages are what we might call the creative kinds of language, not just "ooh" and "ah" with calling and warning cries, but a meaningful language. In this way, by forging linguistic communication of ever increasing precision and subtlety, man must gradually have become a self-conscious being aware of his own identity or selfhood.

Following Popper we can believe that man made himself through the World 3 that he was making, which in the earlier stages must have been largely his linguistic development. We have to explain the fantastically rapid evolutionary change whereby the brain grew from the 600 cm^3 of *Australopithecus* about 1.7 million years ago to the full human size of 1500 cm^3 some 100,000 years ago. A developing language with its *descriptive and argumentative functions* (Popper) would give immense selective advantages to primitive men, first in their welding together in tribes and second in their communal grouping for hunting and fighting. Progressive cerebral development would be necessary for the progressive linguistic development. No doubt tool culture also helped because this was dependent on cerebral development for the skilled control of movements. So we have the concept that man was growing himself through culture by a kind of cross-catalysis. Through the earliest hominids and into the lower Paleolithic there was initially a very slow advance in brain and culture, then gradually there came progressive acceleration until the great cultural advances of the upper Paleolithic.

The more recent development of Paleolithic man is exemplified for us by the Lascaux cave paintings. Such artistic representation of animals could only have been done by a kind of early art school operating by linguistic description and criticism. Language must already have been a highly developed form of communication between those cooperating in such artistic achievements in which the forms and movements of animals had to be visualized and remembered and graphically represented. Following Popper, my theme is that in this long Paleolithic era of hundreds of millennia man was creating himself in all aspects of World 2 by creating his culture, the World 3 of Fig. 6-1. These double processes of creation are indissolubly locked together, and are linked with brain growth.

The progressive acceleration of cultural development can be attributed to a progressive skill and effectiveness in linguistic communication and the consequent development of technology that distinguishes the Neolithic age from the relatively slow development of the long Paleolithic era. Thence came the Mesopotamian and Egyptian civilizations which mark the origins of our time. We are still in this acceleration, at least in some aspects of our culture. For example, look at the output of scientific papers. We don't know what to do about this accelerating volume. In the earlier days, cultural advance was a thousand times slower, even hundreds of thousands times slower than today. In those maturing civilizations of the near east the exigencies of survival were no longer dominant in the thoughts of men and the creative imagination of man could instead be expressed in literature, in art, in architecture, and in the further developments in religion, in philosophy, and in science that are associated with his attempts to understand the manner of being he was, his origin, and his destiny.

It must be recognized that each human individual has to be educated from babyhood to be able to participate even at the simplest level in the culture he has been born into, though of course he carries genetically the potentiality for this participation. This generalization applies to babies from all races. Their cultural development either into the Stone Age culture of primitive men of today into which they may be born or to that of the advanced technological cultures is dependent on their opportunities to learn. A very young child from a Stone Age culture can be assimilated readily to our culture, its achievement being of course dependent on what we may call "brain potentiality"; and, conversely, a very young child of our culture, if immersed in a Stone Age culture, would carry no genetic memory whatsoever of our culture and would merely accept the primitive culture of that society with its tremendous cultural impoverishment without any inkling of its proper birthright.

Everyone in his own lifetime has to recapitulate the whole sequence of cultural development of mankind, more or less. We do not start off making stone axes, but we have to start off with primitive toys and language and work up from there. Also, we start with primitive behavior patterns, and one measure of civilization is the development of civilized behavior. The brain is fully developed by genetic instructions, even the speech areas being built in readiness for the learning of language, but all of culture has to be learned, which we can assume is by the growth of microstructures as suggested in Chap. 5. This is the exciting challenge of human existence—that we are born with immense potentialities. The human brain has evolved in this amazing process of cross-catalysis with cultural performance in a way which we still do not properly understand. How did it come that mathematical geniuses evolved just to survive in a jungle? Evidently more understanding is required!

There is much misunderstanding and downright error in popular beliefs today that environment is dominant in the creation of intelligence. It can be stated quite categorically that brains are built by the complex processes resulting from genetic endowment and all the secondary instructions deriving therefrom in fetal life (cf. Chap. 5). At that stage maternal malnutrition or infection or toxemia may have a deleterious effect. But the essential building of the brain with all its wonderful and various potentialities is complete soon after birth. Geniuses are born, not made. But they have to find the particular métier that matches their exquisite brain potentiality. If this happens, you have a Mozart or Mendelsohn or a Keats with their marvelous youthful creativity; and in our own days Bobby Fischer at age 6 discovered that he had been born with the brain of a chess genius. We still are gravely underestimating the tremendous range in the brain performances apart altogether from environmental influences. The environment is important simply for discovering and using what we have inherited. This is the essence of the age-old nature-nurture problem.

THE HUMAN PERSON

In this last section we will consider the conscious self that we have seen is central to all the conscious experiences of World 2 (Fig. 6-2). This is the personal uniqueness that each of us knows only for himself. This uniqueness has come to us, to each of us in our own lifetime. It is something that we know about only in ourselves. We can talk about it to others if we wish, but they cannot experience any of our World 2. It is private to us. This personal uniqueness and all aspects of its associated experiences are dependent upon the brain; yet it is not entirely dependent on the genetic instructions that built the brain in the manner that is still only vaguely understood (Chap. 5). I believe that my genetic coding is not responsible for my uniqueness as an experiencing being, as I have argued in my book *Facing Reality*. Of course, I have a unique genetic coding, as indeed do all of us who do not have an identical twin, but the probability of the existence of such a unique code is fantastically low: even 1 in $10^{10,000}$. Thus the theory that the uniqueness of the code is the determinant of the uniqueness of the self results in such inconceivable improbabilities that it cannot be an explanation. Nor do my postnatal experiences and education provide a satisfactory explanation of the uniqueness of the self that I experience. It is a necessary but not a sufficient condition.

We do not know how we came to be this unique self that is tied into our brain in a way we do not understand and as is diagrammatically shown in Figs. 6-3 and 6-17. We go through life living with this mysterious existence of ourselves as experiencing beings. I believe that we have to accept what I call a personalist philosophy—that central to our experienced existence is our personal uniqueness.

I think that, for my personal life as a conscious self, the brain is necessary, but it is not sufficient. In liaison with the brain events in World 1, there is the World 2 of my conscious experience, including a personal self at the core of my being. Throughout our lifetime this personal self has continuity despite the failure of liaison with the brain in states of unconsciousness such as dreamless sleep, anesthesia, coma. The brain states are then unsuitable for liaison, but the self can achieve in dreams a partial liaison in the brain states of *REM sleep*. Thus there is evidence that the self in World 2 has an autonomous existence, bridging gaps of unconsciousness when the brain fails to be in a state of liaison. The ultimate question is: What happens when at death the brain disintegrates and the self has permanently lost its instrument of liaison? I evade an answer by stating that there are two linked mysteries in our existence as self-conscious beings: coming-to-be and ceasing-to-be. Together they constitute the same existential problems. I believe that there is meaning to be discovered in this personal life of ours. I believe that we have to live life as if it is a great adventure, and I believe that we have to recognize this for all others. Each human being is a person with this mysterious conscious self associated with his brain. He develops his brain potentialities from his lifetime of learning various aspects of World 3, and so becomes a cultured and civilized human being. It is the World 2 $\rightleftharpoons$ World 3 interaction in all its various intensity and richness that distinguishes a human being from other animals that we can regard as "things." Without that interaction you could be a thing and you could be good material for Skinner with his *Beyond Freedom and Dignity*! But I believe that as human beings we have freedom and dignity. Skinner's theory and the technique of operant conditioning were developed from his experiments on pigeons and rats. Let them be the beneficiaries!

I wish to close with a brief quotation from the end of my book *Facing Reality* where I give some of the thoughts appropriate for the conclusion of this book in which the theme ascends from simple neurobiological levels through to the human brain and ultimately to the mystery of the relationship of the brain to human self-consciousness and cultural achievements. "Because of the mystery of our being as unique self-conscious existences, we can have hope as we set our own soft sensitive and fleeting personal experience against the terror and immensity of illimitable space and time. Are we not participants in the meaning where there is else no meaning? Do we not experience and delight in fellowship, joy, harmony, truth, love and beauty where there else is only the mindless universe?"

REFERENCES

Andersen, P., and S. A. Andersson (1968): *Physiological Basis of the Alpha Rhythm*, Appleton, New York.

Dimond, S. J., and J. G. Beaumont (eds.) (1974): *Hemisphere Function in the Human Brain*, Wiley, New York.

Dobzhansky, T. (1962): *Mankind Evolving: The Evolution of the Human Species*, Yale University Press, New Haven.

Eccles, J. C. (1953): *The Neurophysiological Basis of Mind: The Principles of Neurophysiology*, Clarendon Press, Oxford.

Eccles, J. C. (1958): "The Physiology of Imagination," *Sci. Amer.*, 1958; reprinted in *Altered States of Awareness*, Freeman, San Francisco, 1972, pp. 31–40.

Eccles, J. C. (1970): *Facing Reality: Philosophical Adventures by a Brain Scientist*, Springer, New York.

Eccles, J. C. (1973): "Brain, Speech and Consciousness," *Naturwissenschaften*, 60:167–176.

Feigl, H. (1967): *The "Mental" and the "Physical,"* University of Minnesota Press, Minneapolis.

Gazzaniga, M. S. (1967): "The Split Brain in Man," *Sci. Amer.*, 1967; reprinted in *Physiological Psychology*, Freeman, San Francisco, 1971, pp. 118–123.

Gazzaniga, M. S., J. E. Bogen, and R. W. Sperry (1965): "Observations on Visual Perception after Disconnexion of the Cerebral Hemispheres in Man," *Brain*, 88:221–236.

Geschwind, N. (1972): "Language and the Brain," *Sci. Amer.*, 226:76–83.

Geschwind, N. (1974): "The Anatomical Basis of Hemispheric Differentiation," in S. J. Dimond and J. G. Beaumont (eds.), *Hemisphere Function in the Human Brain*, Wiley, New York, pp. 7–24.

Geschwind, N., and W. Levitsky (1968): "Human Brain: Left-Right Asymmetries in Temporal Speech Region," *Science*, **161**:186–187.

Hécaen, H. (1967): "Brain Mechanisms Suggested by Studies of Parietal Lobes," in C. H. Millikan and F. L. Darley (eds.), *Brain Mechanisms Underlying Speech and Language*, Grune & Stratton, New York and London, pp. 146–166.

Hubel, D. H. (1963): "The Visual Cortex of the Brain," *Sci. Amer.*, 1963; reprinted in *From Cell to Organism*, Freeman, San Francisco, 1967, pp. 54–62.

Hubel, D. H., and T. Wiesel (1962): "Receptive Fields, Binocular Interaction and Functional Architecture in the Cat's Visual Cortex," *J. Physiol.*, **160**:106–154.

Jones, E. G., and T. P. S. Powell (1970): "An Anatomical Study of Converging Sensory Pathways within the Cerebral Cortex of the Monkey," *Brain*, **93**:793–820.

Kety, S. S. (1970): "The Biogenic Amines in the Central Nervous System: Their Possible Roles in Arousal, Emotion, and Learning," in F. O. Schmitt (ed.), *Neurosciences*, Rockefeller University Press, New York, pp. 324–336.

Levy-Agresti, J., and R. W. Sperry (1968): "Differential Perceptual Capacities in Major and Minor Hemispheres," *Proc. Nat. Acad. Sci. U.S.*, **61**:1151.

Levy, J. (1974): "Psychological Implications of Bilateral Asymmetry," in S. J. Dimond and J. G. Beaumont (eds.), *Hemisphere Function in the Human Brain*, Wiley, New York, pp. 121–183.

Levy, J., C. Trevarthen, and R. W. Sperry (1972): "Perception of Bilateral Chimeric Figures Following Hemispheric Deconnexion," *Brain*, **95**:61–78.

Libet, B. (1966): "Brain Stimulation and the Threshold of Conscious Experience," in J. C. Eccles (ed.), *Brain and Conscious Experience*, Springer, New York.

Milner, B. (1967): "Brain Mechanisms Suggested by Studies of Temporal Lobes," in C. H. Millikan and F. L. Darley (eds.), *Brain Mechanisms Underlying Speech and Language*, Grune & Stratton, New York and London, pp. 122–145.

Milner, B. (1974): "Hemispheric Specialization: Scope and Limits," in F. O. Schmitt and F. G. Worden (eds.), *The Neurosciences: Third Study Program*, MIT Press, Cambridge, pp. 75–89.

Mountcastle, V. B. (1967): "The Problem of Sensing and the Neural Coding of Sensory Events," in G. C. Quarton, T. Melnechuk, and F. O. Schmitt (eds.), *The Neurosciences*, Rockefeller University Press, New York, pp. 393–408.

Penfield, W., and H. Jasper (1954): *Epilepsy and the Functional Anatomy of the Human Brain*, Little, Brown, Boston.

Penfield, W., and L. Roberts (1959): *Speech and Brain Mechanisms*, Princeton University Press, Princeton, N.J.

Polten, E. P. (1973): *Critique of the Psycho-Physical Identity Theory*, Mouton, The Hague.

Popper, K. R. (1972): *Objective Knowledge—An Evolutionary Approach*, Clarendon Press, Oxford.

Popper, K. R., and J. C. Eccles (1976): *The Self and its Brain*, Springer-Verlag, Heidelberg, London.

Ratliff, F. (1972): "Contour and Contrast," *Sci. Amer.*, **226**:91–101 (Mach Bands).

Sherrington, C. S. (1940): *Man on His Nature*, Cambridge University Press, Cambridge and London.

Sperry, R. W. (1964): "The Great Cerebral Commissure," *Sci. Amer.*, **210**:42–52.
Sperry, R. W. (1968): "Hemisphere Deconnection and Unity of Conscious Awareness," *Amer. Psychol.*, **23**:723–733.
Sperry, R. W. (1969): "A Modified Concept of Consciousness," *Psychol. Rev.*, **76**:532–536.
Sperry, R. W. (1970a): "Perception in the Absence of the Neocortical Commissures," in *Perception and Its Disorders*, Res. Publ. A.R.N.M.D., vol. 48, The Association for Research in Nervous and Mental Disease.
Sperry, R. W. (1970b): "Cerebral Dominance in Perception," in F. A. Young and D. B. Lindsley (eds.), *Early Experience in Visual Information Processing in Perceptual and Reading Disorders*, Nat. Acad. Sci., Washington, D.C.
Sperry, R. W. (1974): "Lateral Specialization in the Surgically Separated Hemispheres," in F. O. Schmitt and F. G. Worden (eds.), *The Neurosciences: Third Study Program*, MIT Press, Cambridge, pp. 5–19.
Szentágothai, J. (1969): "Architecture of the Cerebral Cortex," in H. H. Jasper, A. A. Ward, and A. Pope (eds.), *Basic Mechanisms of the Epilepsies*, Little, Brown, Boston, pp. 13–28.
Wada, J. A., R. J. Clarke, and A. E. Hamm (1973): "Morphological Asymmetry of Temporal and Frontal Speech Zones in Human Cerebral Hemispheres: Observations on 100 Adult and 100 Infant Brains," *Xth Int. Cong. Neurol.*, Barcelona.
Zaidel, E. (1976): "Auditory Language Comprehension in the Right Hemisphere Following Cerebral Commisurotomy and Hemispherectomy: A Comparison with Child Language and Aphasia," in E. Zurif and A. Caramazza (eds.), *The Acquisition and Breakdown of Language: Parallels and Divergencies,* John Hopkins Press, Baltimore.

General References

Adrian, E. D. (1947): *The Physical Background of Perception*, Clarendon Press, Oxford.

Akert, K., and P. G. Waser (eds.) (1969): *Mechanisms of Synaptic Transmission Progress in Brain Research*, vol. 31, Elsevier, Amsterdam.

Andersen, P., and J. K. S. Jansen (eds.) (1970): *Excitatory Synaptic Mechanisms*, Universitetsforlaget, Oslo.

Bodian, D. (1967): "Neurons, Circuits, and Neuroglia," in G. C. Quarton, T. Melnechuk, and F. O. Schmitt (eds.), *The Neurosciences*, Rockefeller University Press, New York, pp. 6–24.

Brodal, A. (1969): *Neurological Anatomy*, Oxford University Press, New York.

Buser, P., and M. Imbert (1975): *Neurophysiologie Fonctionelle*, Hermann, Paris, 465 pp.

Cole, K. S. (1968): *Membranes, Ions and Impulses*, University of California Press, Berkeley and Los Angeles.

De Robertis, E. (1975): *Synaptic Receptors: Isolation and Molecular Biology*, Marcel Dekker, New York, 387 pp.

Dimond, S. J., and J. G. Beaumont (eds.) (1974): *Hemisphere Function in the Human Brain*, Wiley, New York.

Doty, R. W. (1970): "The Brain," in *Britannica Yearbook of Science and the Future*, Encyclopedia Britannica (W. Benton, publisher), Chicago.

Eccles, J. C. (1953): *The Neurophysiological Basis of Mind: The Principles of Neurophysiology*, Clarendon Press, Oxford.

Eccles, J. C. (1957): *The Physiology of Nerve Cells*, The Johns Hopkins Press, Baltimore.

Eccles, J. C. (1964): *The Physiology of Synapses*, Springer, Göttingen, Berlin, and Heidelberg.

Eccles, J. C. (ed.) (1966): *Brain and Conscious Experience*, Springer, Heidelberg.

Edds, M. V., D. S. Barkley, and D. M. Fambrough (1972): "Genesis of Neuronal Patterns," *Neurosci. Res. Prog. Bull.*, **10**:254–367.

von Euler, C., S. Skoglund, and U. Soderberg (eds.) (1968): *Structure and Function of Inhibitory Neuronal Mechanisms*, Pergamon, Oxford.

Granit, R. (1955): *Receptors and Sensory Perception*, Yale University Press, New Haven.

Hubbard, J. I. (ed.) (1974): *The Peripheral Nervous System*, Plenum, New York and London.

Karczmar, A., and J. C. Eccles (eds.) (1972): *Brain and Human Behavior*, Springer, New York, Heidelberg, and Berlin.

Kuffler, S. W., and J. G. Nicolls (1976): *From Neuron to Brain: A Cellular Approach to the Function of the Nervous System*, Sinauer, Sunderland, Mass.

Mountcastle, V. B. (1975): "The View from Within: Pathways to the Study of Perception," *The Johns Hopkins Medical Journal*, **136**:109–131.

Palay, S. L. (1967): "Principles of Cellular Organization in the Nervous System," in G. C. Quarton, T. Melnechuk, and F. O. Schmitt (eds.), *The Neurosciences*, Rockefeller University Press, New York, pp. 24–31.

Pappas, G. D., and D. P. Purpura (eds.) (1972): *Structure and Function of Synapse*, Raven Press, New York, 308 pp.

Perkel, D. H., and T. H. Bullock (1968): "Neural Coding," *Neurosci. Res. Progr. Bull.*, **6**:221–348.

Popper, K. R., and J. C. Eccles (1976): *The Self and its Brain*, Springer-Verlag, Heidelberg, London.

Schmidt, R. F. (ed.) (1972): *Grundrissder Neurophysiologie*, Springer, Berlin, Heidelberg, New York, 315 pp.

Sherrington, C. S. (1906): *The Integrative Action of the Nervous System*, Yale University Press, New Haven.

Sholl, D. A. (1956): *The Organization of the Cerebral Cortex*, Methuen, London, and Wiley, New York.

Young, J. Z. (1960): *A Model of the Brain*, Clarendon Press, Oxford.

Glossary

Acetylcholine (ACh)   A simple organic molecule: acetic acid + choline (Fig. 2-10B).

Acetylcholine esterase (AChE)   An enzyme splitting ACh into acetic acid and choline (Figs. 1-12, 2-10B).

Action potential   See Impulse (Figs. 1-7, 1-8, 1-11, 1-16).

Adenosine triphosphatase (ATPase)   An enzyme splitting off phosphate from ATP and so producing energy.

Adenosine triphosphate (ATP)   A rich energy-producing nucleotide.

Afferent fibers   Nerve fibers conveying impulses into the brain (Figs. 1-6, 3-13).

All-or-nothing   As illustrated in Fig. 1-11, a stimulus either setting up a full-size impulse or nothing.

Alpha motoneurons   The large motoneurons innervating contractile muscle (Fig. 2-1).

Alpha rhythm   A rhythmic electrical potential recorded from the surface of the brain; see Fig. 6-7.

Amacrine cells   Special inhibitory cells in the retina.

Amino acid   An organic acid with an NH_2 group.

Amnestic syndrome   Loss of all memory except short-term memory.

Annulospiral ending   A receptor located in a special part of a muscle (the muscle spindle, cf. Fig. 4-7). It signals stretch of a muscle (Figs. 1-8*A*, 3-1*A*, 4-7).

Anticholinesterase   A substance preventing the action of the enzyme acetylcholine esterase.

Archicortex   The ancient part of the cerebral cortex such as the hippocampus.

Association cortex   That part of neocortex that is not a primary receiving or transmitting area (Figs. 4-1, 4-15, 4-16, 4-17, 4-18).

Astroglia   A special variety of glial cells (see glia).

Autocatalyze   A self-stimulating action of positive feedback.

Axo-axonic synapses   Axon terminals making synapses on axons; see Fig. 3-12.

Axon   A nerve fiber; the principal branch from a nerve cell (Figs. 1-3, 1-4*A*, 1-6, 1-11, 1-15, 1-16, 1-18, 1-19).

Axon, giant   Very large nerve fibers as in Fig. 1-10.

Axon-trailing method   Suggested manner of synaptic connection when cell migrates, as with Purkinje cells in Fig. 5-1*B*.

Axon transport   Flow of specific chemical substances along an axon.

Axoplasmic flow   As for axon transport (cf. Figs. 5-14, 5-15).

Azide   An enzyme poison, preventing oxidation in the cell.

Basal ganglia   Large collections of neurons deep to the cerebral cortex (Fig. 4-17).

Basket cells   Inhibitory cells in the cerebellar cortex (Fig. 4-11, BC) and in the hippocampus (Fig. 3-10*Fb*).

Bergmann glia   A special variety of glia in the cerebellum, running vertically through the cerebellar cortex.

Bicuculline   A convulsant alkaloid extracted from plants that powerfully blocks GABA action at synapses.

Blood-brain barrier   A protective encapsulation of blood vessels in the brain which prevents the diffusion to the neurons of the brain of many substances in the blood, particularly those with large molecules.

Botulinum toxin   A powerful bacterial toxin that prevents the liberation of acetylcholine from nerve terminals on muscle.

Boutons   Synaptic knobs.

Brain-mind problem   The important scientific-philosophical problem which is concerned with the reciprocal action between brain events and mental events.

Cable transmission   Transmission of a potential charge along a nerve fiber in the manner of an electric cable and not as an impulse.

Cartridge type of synapse   A special complex synapse on dendrites of pyramidal cells; see Fig. 4-6.

Central reflex pathway   Any simple nervous pathway traversing the central nervous system, usually employed for spinal reflexes (cf. Figs. 1-6, 3-1*A*).

Cerebellar nuclei   Collections of nerve cells deep in the cerebellum that mediate the output from the cerebellar Purkinje cells; see Fig. 4-11 (CN).

Cerebello-spinal connectivities   See Fig. 4-20.

Cerebro-cerebellar pathways   Complex pathways linking the cerebral cortex and the cerebellum in both directions; see Figs. 4-14, 4-15, 4-16.

Chemical specification   Specific chemical structures on the surface of nerve fibers and nerve cells that control the development of connectivities (Fig. 1-12).

Choline acetyl transferase   An enzyme that is responsible for the synthesis of acetylcholine from choline and acetic acid (Fig. 2-10B).

Cholinesterase   An enzyme that breaks acetylcholine down into choline and acetic acid (Fig. 2-10B).

Climbing fibers   Afferent fibers to the cerebellar cortex arising from the inferior olive and climbing around the dendrites of Purkinje cells; CF in Fig. 4-11.

Clones   The assemblage of cells made by successive subdivisions of an initial parent cell (Figs. 5-1A,5-5A).

Coactivation   The simultaneous activation of alpha and gamma motoneurons (Fig. 4-8).

Cognitive experience   A conscious thought or experience.

Collaginase   An enzyme that acts on and destroys the collagen fibers (connective tissue).

Collaterals   Branches of nerve axons in the central nervous system (Figs. 3-9, 3-10, 3-11).

Complex and hypercomplex cells   Names given to cells in the visual cortex surrounding the primary visual cortex that exhibit sensitivity to special spatial properties of the retinal stimulation.

Conditioned reflex   A reflex response which is developed in special training procedures.

Conjunction theory of learning   Learning is attributed to the growth of synapses resulting from conjunction of a special synaptic input (the instructional input) with the testing synaptic input.

Corpus callosum   The tract of nerve fibers connecting the cerebral hemispheres; see Figs. 6-11, 6-12.

Cortex, cerebral   The thin outer layer of grey matter that covers the whole folded surface of the cerebral hemispheres (Fig. 1-2).

Cuneate nucleus   Relay nucleus on the main afferent pathway from forelimb receptors to the brain; see Fig. 3-13.

Cuneo-cerebellar tract   The pathway from the cuneate nucleus terminating as mossy fibers in the cerebellum.

Curare   A drug extracted from South American plants that paralyzes nerve muscle transmission by occupying acetylcholine receptor sites (Fig. 2-3E).

Cutaneous mechanoreceptors   See receptor organs, tactile.

Dale's principle   The same transmitter substance is liberated from all synaptic endings made by any particular nerve cell.

Decomposition of movement   A disorder of movement resulting from cerebellar lesions in which the patient has to move each joint separately.

Deiters' nucleus   A collection of large nerve cells in the brainstem that is acted on by vestibular and cerebellar output and whose axons travel down the spinal cord as the vestibulospinal tract; DN in Fig. 4-20.

Dendrites   Large and often complex branches of nerve cells that receive synapses from other nerve cells; see Figs. 1-2B, 1-3, 1-4A, 4-6, 4-11.

Dendritic spine synapses   Synapses formed on the numerous spines of dendrites; see Figs. 1-3B, 5-19.

Dendrodendritic synapses   Synapses that are formed in special situations between dendrites; see Fig. 3-15.

Deoxyribonucleic acid (DNA)   The very large complex organic molecules in double helix array that are the basis of genetic coding.

Depolarization   The diminution of the normal resting potential across a membrane.

Differentiating mitosis   Cell divisions in which the daughter cells have an effectively different genetic coding from the parents (Figs. 5-1, 5-5).

Dinitrophenol   An organic substance that poisons oxidative enzymes.

Disinhibition   The removal or reduction of background inhibition; it effectively acts as an excitation.

Dominant hemisphere   The cerebral hemisphere responsible for linguistic and ideational performance; see Figs. 6-12, 6-17, 6-18.

Dorsal column nuclei   The collections of nerve cells which relay the main pathways up the spinal cord via the dorsal columns to the brain (cf. cuneate nucleus, Fig. 3-13).

Dorsal spinocerebellar tract   The main pathway conveying cutaneous and muscle sense up the spinal cord to the cerebellum where it ends as mossy fibers (DSCT in Figs. 4-14, 4-20).

Dualist   One who believes in the separate existence of material and mental events; cf. Fig. 6-2.

Dynamic engram   Neuronal organization in the brain which depends on specific patterning of impulse transmissions, which endures even for hours and which exists only by virtue of this continued patterned performance.

Dyslexia   Reading disability.

Edrophonium   A substance which very powerfully and repetitively depresses acetylcholine esterase (Fig. 2-5D).

Electrical synapse   A synapse in which the transmission is due to the flow of electrical currents and not to specific chemical action.

Electrochemical gradient   The value representing the voltage across a membrane for a particular charged particle, being compounded of the electrochemical potential for that particle and the voltage gradient across the membrane (see Fig. 1-13).

Electrochemical potential   Derived by the Nernst equation from the logarithmic relationship of the concentrations of the charged particles on either side of a membrane (Fig. 1-13A).

Electroencephalogram   Electrical potentials recorded from the surface of the brain that are generated by activity in the brain (see Fig. 6-7).

Electrophoretic injection   The injection of charged particles (ions) out of a pipette by an applied current (Figs. 2-4, 2-9).

Endplate potential (EPP)   The potential change generated across an endplate membrane of muscle by a nerve impulse; see Fig. 2-3C.

Endplate potential, miniature (min EPP)   The unitary components of the endplate potential generated by the quantal discharge of transmitter from the nerve ending (Figs. 2-5, 2-6).

Engram   A patterned arrangement of neuronal connections via synapses that have been given increased effectiveness in learning.

Ependyma   The thin membrane composed of cells on the surface of the cerebral ventricle; see Fig. 5-1.

Equilibrium potential The membrane potential at which there is equivalent movement of charged particles in both directions across the membrane. Also used for processes depending on charged particle movement such as the EPP, EPSP, and IPSP (E_{EPSP} and E_{IPSP} in Fig. 3-3 and E_{EPP} in Fig. 2-3B).

Evolving movement Descriptive term of any ongoing movement, that of a limb, for example, Figs. 4-16, 4-20).

Excitatory postsynaptic potential (EPSP) The membrane potential generated by excitatory synaptic action (Figs. 3-2, 3-3C).

Excitatory synapses Synapses in which the transmitter normally acts to depolarize the postsynaptic membrane and so to excite the postsynaptic cell; see Figs. 1-4B, 1-5, 2-14C, 3-7C.

Expectancy wave A potential change recorded from the surface of the brain and which arises in anticipation of a conditioned movement.

Extensor muscle A muscle which acts to straighten a joint (Fig. 3-1A).

External germinal layer A layer of cells (germinal cells) formed on the surface of the developing cerebellum and which generates many cell types of the cerebellum [Figs. 5-1B, 5-2 (MU), 5-6.]

Extrafusal fibers The ordinary muscle fibers responsible for the contractions of muscles, distinguished from intrafusal fibers of muscle spindles (Fig. 4-7).

Extrasynaptic The surface membrane that is not covered by synapses.

Fastigial nucleus One of the cerebellar nuclei that is responsible for transmission out of the cerebellum; FN in Fig. 4-20.

Flexor muscles Muscles producing bending of joints (Fig. 3-1A).

Flexor reflexes Activate flexor muscles (Fig. 1-6B).

Frequency potentiation The increased action of synapses when repetitively stimulated at high frequencies (Fig. 5-16B, C).

Gamma-amino-butyric acid (GABA) An amino acid that is the inhibitory transmitter substance in many central synapses.

Gamma loop The operative path employing gamma fibers and gamma motoneurons in movement control: gamma motoneurons, muscle spindles, Ia fibers, alpha motoneurons, extrafusal muscle contraction; see Fig. 4-7.

Gamma motoneurons The small motoneurons innervating intrafusal muscle fibers (Fig. 4-7).

Ganglion cell Nerve cells peripheral to the central nervous system. Many relay synaptically to the viscera; see Fig. 2-14.

Gap junction The very close approximation of the presynaptic and postsynaptic membranes that characterizes electrically transmitting synapses.

Genone The collective name given to the operative DNA of a cell.

Germinal cells Cells which in embryonic development give rise to neuroblasts and hence nerve cells (GC in Fig. 5-5).

Glia (glial cells) Nonneuronal cells in the central nervous system that perform a multitude of ancillary functions: oligodendroglia, astroglia.

Glutamate Derived from the diacidic amino acid, glutamic acid.

Glutaraldehyde A substance used in fixation of nerve tissue in order to distinguish between excitatory and inhibitory synapses by vesicular shape; see Fig. 1-4B.

Glycine An amino acid that acts as an inhibitory transmitter in many central synapses.

Golgi cells Special cells in the cerebellar cortex that act to give widespread inhibition; see Fig. 4-11 (GC).

Granule cells Immensely numerous small cells in the cerebellar cortex [Fig. 4-11 (GrC)].

Growth theory of learning Learning is attributed to the growth of specific synapses resulting in preferred neuronal pathways in the brain (Fig. 5-19B, C).

Habituation A progressive diminution of reflex responses that are repetitively elicited.

Heterotypic regeneration Regeneration in which the vacated synaptic sites are occupied by presynaptic fibers different from the original fibers (Fig. 5-12).

Hippocampus A special part of the cerebral cortex (the archicortex); see Figs. 1-3B, 3-10.

Homotypic regeneration Regeneration in which the vacated synaptic sites are occupied by presynaptic fibers similar to the original fibers (Fig. 5-13).

Horizontal cells Special inhibitory cells in the retina.

Hydrophilic Water-attractive.

Hyperpolarization The increased potential produced across a cell membrane.

Hypothalamus A deep-lying part of the brain concerned in visceral control, for example, in relation to temperature, salt, water, food, endocrines, and mood.

Impulse A message traveling as a brief action potential in nerve or muscle fibers (Figs. 1-7, 1-8, 1-11, 1-16).

Inferior frontal convolution Area of the anterior speech cortex (Broca); see Fig. 6-8.

Inferior olive Nucleus in brainstem responsible for origin of climbing fibers to cerebellum (IO, Figs. 4-14, 4-15, 4-20).

Inhibitory neurons Neurons (nerve cells) exclusively responsible for inhibitory synaptic action (Figs. 3-9, 3-10, 3-11).

Inhibitory pathways Pathways composed of the axons of inhibitory neurons.

Inhibitory postsynaptic potential (IPSP) The membrane potential produced by activation of inhibitory synapses, normally hyperpolarization (Figs. 3-6, 3-7).

Inhibitory synapses Special synapses (Fig. 1-4B) made by inhibitory cells and concerned in producing IPSPs.

Inner sense See Fig. 6-2.

Intermediate-term memory Memories having a duration of seconds to hours and are believed to be due to increased synaptic efficacy (Figs. 5-17, 5-18).

Interneuron Excitatory or inhibitory nerve cells in the central nervous system which usually have a short range of action; see Figs. 1-6B, 3-1A, 4-6, 4-11.

Interpositus nucleus One of the cerebellar nuclei that is responsible for transmission out of the cerebellum; IP in Fig. 4-14.

Intrafusal fibers The small muscle fibers in muscle spindles (Fig. 4-7).

Isotonic Physiological solutions which have the same osmotic pressure as normal extracellular fluids.

Lateral geniculate body The main relay station from the eye to the visual cortex (Fig. 6-4A).

Lateral reticular nucleus (LRN) A relay nucleus for pathways to the cerebellum that end as mossy fibers (Figs. 4-14, 4-20).

Liaison brain   That special part of the brain postulated to be in liaison with conscious experience (Figs. 6-2, 6-3, 6-17).

Limbic lobe   The collective name given to the many nuclei and associated structures that originate in the primitive olfactory (smell) brain, particularly the hippocampus and related structures.

Membrane   The very delicate structure constituting the surface of cells; see Fig. 1-12.

Membrane potential   The electrical potential across the cell membrance; see Figs. 1-11, 1-13, 3-3.

Memory, long-term   Enduring memories from hours to a lifetime, presumably with a structural base (see engram).

Memory, short-term   Fleeting memories of seconds duration, presumably with a patterned impulse base (see dynamic engram).

Microelectrodes   Fine conductors insulated except for their tips, either of glass with a tip diameter of the order of a micron or so filled with a conducting salt solution, or of metal coated with insulation except at the tip.

Minor hemisphere   The nonlinguistic hemisphere, almost always the right (Figs. 6-9, 6-12), with special performances listed in Fig. 6-18.

Mitochondria   Special organelles in cells with enzymes concerned with the provision of energy by oxidation; see Figs. 1-4*B*, 2-2*B*.

Mitotic competency   Ability of cells to divide by mitosis.

Mitotic divisions   Cell divisions depending on mitosis and normally forming clones, as in Figs. 5-1*A*, 5-5*A*.

Mitral cells   Nerve cells in the olfactory bulb (Fig. 3-15*A*).

Modifiable synapses   Synapses postulated to be changed in their effectiveness by use and disuse (Fig. 5-19).

Mossy fibers   Afferent fibers ending in the cerebellar cortex; see MF in Fig. 4-11.

Motoneurons   Large neurons in the spinal cord and brainstem whose axons innervate muscle fibers; see Figs. 2-1, 3-1, 4-7.

Motor aphasia   Disorder of speech produced by lesion of Broca's area (Fig. 6-8) and characterized by disability to speak, though language is still understood.

Motor cortex   That part of the cerebral cortex concerned directly with the control of movement, the origin of the pyramidal tract; see Figs. 4-1, 4-2.

Motor endplate   The specialized part of the muscle fiber in association with the nerve terminal; see Fig. 2-2*A*.

Motor unit   The unit subserving muscular movement, comprising the motor nerve fiber and muscle fibers innervated thereby; see Fig. 2-1.

Multiple sclerosis   A nervous disease resulting from interruptions of neural pathways to and from the brain as a consequence of degeneration of the myelin sheaths of the nerve fibers in the tracts of the spinal cord.

Muscle spindles   Special encapsulated bundles of fine muscle fibers specially related to muscle stretch receptors; see Fig. 4-7.

Myasthenia gravis   A neurological disease associated with partial paralysis due to defect in nerve-muscle transmission and with extreme fatigability.

Myelin sheath   The laminated wrapping around nerve fibers of membranes composed largely of lipoid molecules; see Fig. 1-19.

Myosin   The contractile protein of muscle fibers.

Neocortex   The most recently developed part of the cerebral cortex composing the cerebral hemispheres; see Figs. 1-1, 1-2, 4-1.

Nerve cell   See neuron.

Nerve fiber   An axon and the principal branch from a nerve cell that may extend for long distances in tracts (central nervous system, Figs. 3-13, 4-2) or in peripheral nerves (Figs. 1-19, 2-1).

Neuroblasts   Special cells that are the precursors of nerve cells, developing directly into them; see Figs. 5-1, 5-5.

Neurofibrils   Fine fibers running along the interior of nerve axons; see Fig. 1-19A.

Neurogenesis   The process whereby nerve cells are made by the sequence of germinal cells to neuroblasts to fully fashioned nerve cells (cf. Figs. 5-1A, 5-5A).

Neuron (nerve cell)   The biological unit of the brain and of the remainder of the nervous system; see Figs. 1-2, 1-3, 1-4, 2-14.

Neuron theory   The theory that the nervous system is composed of individual neurons biologically independent but informationally communicating by synapses.

Neurotubules   Very fine tubules running along the interior of nerve axons.

Nuclei pontis   Nerve cells on the pathway from the cerebral cortex into the cerebellum with axons ending in mossy fibers; NP, Figs. 4-14, 4-15.

Nucleus dentatus   One of the cerebellar nuclei that is responsible for transmission out of the cerebellum to the cerebral cortex (Fig. 4-15).

Nucleus fastigii   See fastigial nucleus.

Olfactory pathway   The pathway for sense of smell passing through the olfactory bulb; see Fig. 3-15.

Optic chiasma   The site of complete (Fig. 5-9A) or partial (Fig. 6-12) crossing of the optic nerves connecting the retina to the brain.

Optic tectum (optic lobe)   In fish and amphibia the part of the brain to which the optic nerves project (Figs. 5-8A, 5-11).

Outer sense   See Fig. 6-2.

Parallel fibers   The multitude of fine fibers running along the molecular layer of the cerebellar folia and making synapses with all the dendrites therein [Figs. 4-11, 4-12, 4-13, 5-3 (PF)].

Pars intermedia   That part of the cerebellar cortex receiving and projecting both to the cerebrum and to the spinal cord [Figs. 4-14, 4-16 (PI)].

Phospholipid   Molecule composed of fatty acid chains and a phosphorylated polar end. The basic structure of cell membranes (Fig. 1-12).

Picrotoxin   A convulsant substance blocking inhibition by GABA.

Positive feedback control   The control by which the output is fed back to give intensification of input.

Posterior speech area of Wernicke   The speech area as evidenced by the effects of lesions causing failure to understand speech; see Fig. 6-8.

Poststimulus time histogram (PSTH)   A plotting of responses that are averaged in small intervals of time after the triggering stimulus.

Postsynaptic membrane   The nerve cell membrane immediately related to the synapse formed by presynaptic fibers ending on it (Figs. 1-4B, 1-5, 2-9D).

Postsynaptic potentiation   The increased synaptic action that follows intensive synaptic stimulation (Figs, 5-17, 5-18).

Presynaptic fibers   The terminal branches of nerve fibers that end as synaptic knobs (Fig. 1-3A).

Presynaptic inhibition The inhibitory action resulting from the depolarization of presynaptic fibers by axo-axonic synapses and the consequent diminution of transmitter output (Fig. 3-12).

Presynaptic inhibitory fibers The fibers which terminate as the axo-axonic synapses responsible for presynaptic inhibition (Fig. 3-12).

Primary afferent fibers The afferent fibers passing from receptor organs into the central nervous system (Figs. 1-6, 3-1, 3-13, 4-7).

Primary reality The experience immediately given in all aspects of consciousness (cf. Fig. 6-2).

Principle of convergence The feature of the nervous system in which many nerve cells project to a single neuron; see Figs. 3-1*B*, 4-11.

Principle of divergence The design feature of the nervous system in which one neuron branches to be distributed widely to other neurons; see Figs. 1-6, 4-11.

Procion yellow A dye used to inject directly into single nerve cells so as to display fully their many dendritic branches and their axons.

Proliferative zone That part of the developing cerebellar cortex in which the germinal cells are dividing; see Fig. 5-6.

Prostigmine A drug powerfully inhibiting acetylcholine esterase (an anticholinesterase) (Fig. 2-3*G*).

Purkinje cells The large cells of the cerebellar cortex whose axons are the sole projecting pathway out of the cortex [Figs. 4-11, 4-12, 4-13, 4-14, 4-15 (PC)].

Pyramidal cells The large pyramidally shaped cells of the cerebral cortex, both neocortex and archicortex, with axons often projecting far from the cell, even down the pyramidal tract (Figs. 1-2*B*, 1-3*B*, 4-2, 4-6, 4-14).

Pyramidal tract The large tract of nerve fibers from the motor cortex down to the motoneurons in the spinal cord. The principal pathway for movement control (Fig. 4-2).

Quantal emission The transmitter emission in packages or quanta from nerve synaptic terminals; occurs either spontaneously or is evoked by nerve impulses (Figs. 2-5, 2-6).

Readiness potential The potential changes recorded from the cerebral cortex during preparatory stages of a voluntary movement (Fig. 4-3).

Receptor organs Structures specialized for transduction from physical or chemical stimuli to nerve impulses. Tactile: mechanoreceptors of skin sensitive to touch or pressure. Light: photoreceptors in retina. Smell: olfactory receptors in nose. Stretch: mechanoreceptors in muscle responsive to stretch or pressure.

Reciprocal synapses Specialized dendrodendritic synaptic structures in the olfactory bulb and retina characterized by reciprocal synaptic action, i.e., excitation in one direction and inhibition in the other (Fig. 3-15).

Red nucleus An important nucleus in the brainstem specially concerned in transmitting the cerebellar output down the spinal cord in the rubrospinal tract [Fig. 4-14 (RN and RST)].

Reflex pathways (reflex arc) Simple neuronal pathways through the central nervous system involving afferent input, various interneuronal linkages, and efferent output by motoneuron discharges (Figs. 1-6, 3-1, 4-7).

Refractory period, absolute The time following a nerve impulse during which it is impossible to generate a second nerve impulse.

Refractory period, relative   The time following the absolute refractory period
during which a stronger stimulus is required to initiate a nerve impulse, the
nerve impulse being smaller and slower (Fig. 1-17).

REM sleep   That phase of sleep characterized by rapid eye movements and that
is usually associated with dreams.

Renshaw cells   Special inhibitory interneurons in the spinal cord that act as a
negative feedback control of motoneurons (Fig. 3-9).

Reticular nucleus   A large, diffuse collection of nerve cells running through the
brainstem, some being concerned in motor control with their tract via the
reticulospinal tract (ReN and ReST of Fig. 4-20).

Reticulospinal tract   See reticular nucleus.

Retinotectal projection   The pathway in amphibians and fish from the retina of
the eye to the tectum; see Fig. 5-8.

Retrograde transport   The transport of substances along nerve axons toward the
cell body in contrast to the usual transport away from the cell body.

Rubrospinal tract   See red nucleus.

Schwann cell   Specialized cells surrounding nerve fibers and forming the myelin
sheath; see Figs. 1-19B,C,D, 2-2.

Secondary endings   The receptor endings on the muscle spindle in addition to the
primary endings or annulospiral endings of Figs. 3-1A and 4-7.

Secondary reality   Knowledge of the external world based upon our experienced
interpretations of our perceptions. See Worlds 1 and 3 of Fig. 6-1.

Selective fasciculation   The growth of nerve fibers along pioneering paths of
earlier similar fibers so that nerve bundles or fascicles are built.

Sensory modality   The distinguishing names of all the various sensations arising
from diverse inputs with their specific receptor organs. See receptor organs.

Septal nuclei   Collections of neurons in the diencephalon that are important relay
centers (Fig. 5-12).

Servoloop control   Automatic control by feedback pathways such as are indicated in the gamma loop of Fig. 4-7.

Servomechanism   Mechanism designed for feedback-control operation.

Soma (cell body)   The expanded part of the nerve cell immediately surrounding
the nucleus and from which branch the dendrites and axons (Fig. 1-3).

Spatial summation   Summation of synaptic actions arising from convergence on
a neuron of pathways coming from different sites (Fig. 3-2J to M).

Specific afferents   Afferent pathways in the brain conveying specific information,
as for example, skin sensation in Figs. 3-13, 3-14 and 4-6 (Spec aff).

Spinal centers   The collective name given to the interneurons and their various
connectivities in the spinal cord.

Stellate cells   Interneurons of a star-shaped character in various parts of the
central nervous system; in the cerebral cortex in Figs. 3-14 and 4-6, and in the
cerebellum in Fig. 4-11 (SC).

Stellate ganglion (squid)   A ganglion characterized by large presynaptic and
postsynaptic fibers (Figs. 1-10A, 2-12H).

Superior temporal convolution   The area of the neocortex forming the center of
the posterior speech cortex of Wernicke (Fig. 6-8).

Synapse   The specialized structure whereby nerve cells communicate, usually by
the specific chemical transmission as in Figs. 1-4, 1-5, 2-2, 2-14C, and 3-7C,
but also electrically by a specially close apposition of membranes.

Synaptic cleft   The narrow space between the pre- and postsynaptic membranes of a chemical synapse (Figs. 1-4B, 1-5, 2-2B, 2-10, 2-11, 2-14C).

Synaptic excitation   Synaptic action depolarizing the postsynaptic membrane and hence tending to generate impulses (Fig. 3-3A,C).

Synaptic inhibition   Synaptic action hyperpolarizing the postsynaptic membrane and hence tending to prevent impulse generation (Fig. 3-3B,D).

Synaptic knob or bouton   The expanded terminal of the presynaptic nerve fiber (Figs. 1-3, 1-4A, 1-5, 3-7C).

Synaptic plasticity   The property of synapses whereby they are changed in functional efficiency, probably by virtue of changes in size (Fig. 5-19).

Synaptic vesicles   Small spherical or ellipsoid organelles in presynaptic nerve terminals that contain packages of transmitter substance (Figs. 1-4B, 1-5, 2-2B, 2-10, 2-11, 2-14C, 3-7C, 3-15B).

Tactile receptors   See receptor organs, tactile.

Tetraethylammonium (TEA)   A substance specifically blocking the gates whereby potassium ions pass through the cell membrane; see Figs. 1-15, 2-11B (K_D).

Tetrodotoxin (TTX)   A substance specifically blocking the gates whereby sodium ions pass through the cell membrane; see Figs. 1-15, 2-11B (Na_D).

Thalamus   The massive collection of nerve cells deep to the cerebral cortex, in part concerned with transmission of cutaneous sense to the cerebrum (Fig. 3-13). (See also ventrolateral thalamus.)

Transneuronal degeneration   The degeneration of nerve cells that occurs when there is degeneration of synapses on their surfaces.

Trialist   One who believes in the existence of three worlds; see Fig. 6-1.

Tritiated leucine (^{3}H-leucine)   The amino acid leucine with partial replacement of hydrogen atoms by radioactive tritium.

Tritiated lysine (^{3}H-lysine)   The amino acid lysine with partial replacement of hydrogen atoms by radioactive tritium.

Tritiated thymidine (^{3}H-thymidine)   Thymidine in which the hydrogen atoms are partly replaced by radioactive tritium.

Trophic influences   Actions from one part of a cell to another or from one cell to another, which are concerned with the growth, maintenance, and metabolism of the cell.

Trophic transport   The postulated mechanism of transport of specific macromolecules within a cell and between cells that is concerned in exerting trophic influences.

Ventrolateral thalamus   That part of the thalamus specially concerned in the transmission from the cerebellum to the cerebrum [Figs. 4-14, 4-15 (VL THAL)].

Vestibulospinal tract   The pathway down the spinal cord from Deiters' nucleus to motoneurons; see Fig. 4-20 (VST).

Visual cortex   That part of the cerebral cortex specially concerned with vision; see Figs. 4-1, 6-4.

Visual field   The area of the surround projecting to the eye and forming an image on the retina; see Fig. 6-12.

World 1   See Fig. 6-1.

World 2   See Fig. 6-1.

World 3   See Fig. 6-1.

Dimensional Abbreviations

DISTANCE

m = meter
cm = centimeter $= 10^{-2}$ m
mm = millimeter $= 10^{-3}$ m
μm = micrometer $= 10^{-6}$ m
A = Angstrom $= 10^{-10}$ m

TIME

s = second
ms = millisecond $= 10^{-3}$ s
μs = microsecond $= 10^{-6}$ s

ELECTRICAL TERMS

Ω = ohm, electrical resistance
MΩ = megaohm $= 10^{6}$ Ω
F = farad, electrical capacity
μF = microfarad $= 10^{-6}$ F
V = volt, electrical potential
mV = millivolt $= 10^{-3}$ V
μV = microvolt $= 10^{-6}$ V
mho = conductance of 1 reciprocal ohm
mmho $= 10^{-3}$ mho
A = ampere, electric current
C = coulomb, electric quantity